Do We Care?

D0165299

Do We Care?

RENEWING CANADA'S COMMITMENT TO HEALTH

proceedings of the first Directions for Canadian Health Care conference

Margaret A. Somerville
Editor

John Ralston Saul

- Richard Cruess • Bob Rae

- Nuala Kenny • Raisa Deber

- Bernard Dickens

McGill-Queen's University Press
Montreal • Kingston • London • Ithaca

©1999 Merck Frosst Canada & Co.

ISBN 0-7735-1877-0 (cloth)
ISBN 0-7735-1878-9 (paper)

Legal deposit first quarter 1999
Bibliothèque nationale du Québec

Printed in Canada

Canadian Cataloguing in Publication Data

Directions for Canadian Health Care Conference (1st: 1998: Toronto, Ont.)
Do we care?: renewing Canada's commitment to health

ISBN 0-7735-1877-0 (bound)
ISBN 0-7735-1878-9 (pbk.)

1. Medical policy — Canada. I. Somerville, Margaret A.-, 1942-   .
II. Saul, John Ralston, 1947-   III. Title

RA449.D57 1999   362.1'0971   C99-900056-X

Book design by Deborah Hodgdon
Page make up by PAGEXPRESS

CONTENTS

ACKNOWLEDGMENTS

Special thanks are in order to Margaret A. Somerville for her dedicated work as Chair of the *Directions for Canadian Health Care* conference; Don Soule, Pierre Paquette and Kevin Skilton at Merck Frosst Canada & Co. for the wonderful idea that sparked both the conference and this book; Susan Usher for chairing the conference planning committee and leading the editorial team at Parkhurst Publishing, which included Owen Dyer and Janalyn Prest; and Robb Beattie for moulding the conference presentations into the following chapters.

INTRODUCTION

Dr. Margaret A. Somerville

The somewhat bland title of the conference this book is based on, *Directions for Canadian Health Care: a framework for sound decisions*, encompasses a highly controversial area of public policy that is of profound importance to all Canadians. I had initially suggested a more dramatic title for the conference, such as "Is Health Policy Killing Canadian Health Care" or "Should We Take Canadian Health Care Off Life-Support," but the other organizers thought that the subject was of sufficient import to not need additional hyperbole.

The fundamental presumption that guided the structuring of the conference and the way the speakers were chosen was that current health policy decisions will have major effects on the quality of our lives well into the future, and that it is essential to make sure that health care reforms fulfill our needs and are compatible with the values our nation is founded on.

While having access to good health care when we are ill is immensely important to each of us, health care is never simply about health care, and certainly not in Canada. Our health care system defines us as communities, as a society, and as a nation. What Canadians are prepared to do, and more importantly, what we are not prepared to do for each other when we are sick, vulnerable, and most in need, says a great deal about Canada, our basic values, and the values that we want to hand on to future generations of Canadians.

Health care is a major force in determining what can be referred to as the ethical and legal tone of a society. For Canada, as for many societies at the end of the 20ᵗʰ century, it is also an extraordinarily important forum in which to work out the principles, attitudes, beliefs, myths and values that will together constitute a new societal paradigm for the decades ahead. This is the "shared story" on which a society is based; the story we narrate, heed, and contribute to in order to form a society. Decisions about health care range from everyday medical and ethical decisions such as providing proper antenatal care to pregnant women or care to dying patients, to decisions about extraordinary new capabilities like reproductive technologies or xenotransplantation (the transplanting of animal organs into humans). These decisions are based on, reflect and form profound individual and societal values.

In short, decisions about health care have a major impact both on the most personal aspects of our lives and on our overall societal structure. There are few, if any, other classes of decisions that have this range of impact. This salient fact means that the health care system functions as the proverbial canary in the societal mine shaft, in terms of testing the ethical air. If the health care canary is sick, we need to be extremely concerned that society itself is facing dangerous times, and that its very coherence and values are at risk.

Most of us agree that our society has an obligation to provide all Canadians with the health care they need. Where we disagree is on how we should fund this, and where we should draw the line between necessary and unnecessary health care. In entering this debate, it is important to recognize that the tone of the debate will be different if one starts from agreement and moves to disagreement, and then, where possible, to consensus, as compared with merely focusing on disagreements. It is very easy to overlook large areas of agreement, especially when the media focus so overwhelmingly on disagreements. Because of this, the "Directions" conference was structured to encourage participants to identify areas of agreement as well as disagreement.

Much of the discussion about health care today has to do with what Dr. Maurice McGregor once called "the costs of our success." We live in an age where medicine has become so successful in achieving its aims, and so specialized, that our society now cannot afford to do everything that it is possible to do for everyone. As a result, a fundamental question of health care has become: How do we deal with allocating those successes? The ongoing discussion surrounding this complex problem often seems to become caught up in what I refer to as the twin dilemmas of "the mouse and the whirlpool." Initially, the discussion takes the shape of a mouse going around faster and faster and faster inside a wheel trying to find a way out, a solution, until the participants end up exhausted and find they have gone nowhere. Then comes the whirlpool, when the discussion's participants start going not only around and around, but also deeper and deeper in ever-narrowing circles. In the end, everyone drowns.

These images sound a warning about the possible outcome of the current health care debate. If this debate is based on despair — as often seems to be the case — rather than hope, it could elicit a nihilistic response which would have an impact on Canadian society that extends far beyond the health care context. The only way to avoid the dangers we are currently facing in this regard is to establish a climate of realistically-based hope and to make a radical shift to new ways of thinking about directions for Canadian health care, and to new ways of feeling about the decisions that we make.

Such change is difficult, even if it is welcome, which it certainly may not be to some decision-makers and participants in the system. As well, people who feel obliged to speak out about the perils and hazards of the current health care system — or the one we seem headed for — may be putting themselves at risk professionally by doing so. In planning the "Directions" conference, the organizers sought out participants with the courage to engage in the health care debate not only on the basis of their knowledge and convictions, but also their imaginations, in order to bring much-needed fresh insight to this debate. This insight is essential if we are to overcome the obstacles we will undoubtedly face in making changes that are necessary and that will ultimately be beneficial.

Another main purpose of the conference was to engage in a transdisciplinary conversation on directions for Canadian health care, and to establish a base that supported continued dialogue of this type. We need a structure to sustain the broad-based, community-level conversations that should go on across this country about the future of health care. In this regard, one of the difficulties has long been the fact that so much of the debate has been dominated by hard-edged economic analysis, which is easy to appreciate and easy to sound authoritative about, especially if you are a politician seeking to win an argument by falling back on apparently irrefutable economic statistics. But while that perspective is essential, it is not sufficient, and so the speakers who addressed economics at the conference were chosen for the breadth of their vision on the role of economics in the health care debate.

Health care is not just a business like any other business. It is not just a matter of statistics and bottom lines. Our decisions about health care must factor in our deepest sense of ourselves, both as individuals and as a society, our most important values and beliefs about the meaning of human life and what it means to be fully human, humane and caring. Moreover, at just the practical level, to engage adequately and competently in a societal conversation about future directions for Canadian health care, we need to take into account a very broad spectrum of perspectives: clinical practice, economics, politics, ethics, and law. The choice of these perspectives and the order in which they are addressed reflect the belief that good health care facts are essential to good ethics in health care, and good medical law depends on good ethics.

We also recognized the need to adopt an integrated approach in exploring these perspectives, one that goes beyond our current multidisciplinary methodologies, which tend to promote the parallel exploration of each perspective. We need to embed these different perspectives in each other in order to take a truly transdisciplinary approach. The main aim of such an approach is to produce integrated knowledge on which we can base important, far-reaching societal decisions such as those involved in fashioning Canada's health care system for the future.

Finally, and most importantly, we realized that our response to the question "What are we doing here (at the "Directions" conference)?", was that we were exploring another question: "Do we care?" This exploration will require us to use all of our human ways of knowing, which John Ralston Saul so eloquently articulates in *The Unconscious Civilization* as including not only reason — our cognitive, logical facility — but also ethics, common sense, intuition, human memory and history, and, above all, imagination and creativity.

SPONSOR'S ADDRESS TO THE CONFERENCE

Merck Frosst Canada & Co. is coming up to its 100th anniversary, a landmark that has our company celebrating the past while considering the future for all Canadians. Today, many of Canada's leading figures in health care policy, notable individuals with expertise across the fields of clinical practice, politics, economics, ethics and law, are gathered here from across the country to discuss one central issue of the utmost importance. Our task over the next two days — to begin building a framework for sound policy in health care.

There is perhaps no other social issue currently more important to Canadians. Virtually every day the citizens of this country read or hear about the stresses and strains on our health care system; some days many of us experience them first-hand as patients. It is not all bad news of course. Yes, there are the horror stories of overcrowded emergency rooms and long waits for elective surgery, but there are also progress reports on new technologies that are saving lives and reducing demands on health care. There are new health professions coming onstream with increasingly sophisticated skills. And most importantly, there is the public, a discerning and informed public that demands a greater measure of choice, access, quality and accountability from the health care system. Our system is indeed evolving to keep pace with the demands of our times, and with the needs of Canadians. But as it does, Canadians need to ensure that it remains a health care system with high standards, a system that balances quality and equality.

Policy forums such as this one are instrumental to the process of change. As we move forward with reforms in health care, I am convinced that the expertise in this room and others like it will help all Canadians by providing the direction needed to balance access, quality and choice; a direction that does not jeopardize the sustainability of our health care system.

Bernard Houde, Vice President, Corporate Affairs,
Merck Frosst Canada & Co.

CHAPTER 1

Health Care at the End of the Twentieth Century

Health Care at the End of the Twentieth Century: Confusing Symptoms For Systems

Dr. John Ralston Saul

When the word "vision" is evoked today, it usually refers to an apparently desperate need for new ideas and new directions to resolve society's fundamental and destructive problems. We regularly advocate abandoning a tired, unfortunate past in order to progress to something entirely new. This tendency to consider only what are perceived to be new solutions is one of our era's most dangerous failings, as it often serves a purpose quite different from solving problems. Over the past half-century, it has consistently served as one of the great mechanisms for taking power: you first convince people that what they have does not work, and second that they therefore need something new. And you just happen to have it.

I am not convinced that there is anything wrong with the fundamental ideas behind Canada's public health system. Medicare's current difficulties derive in part from people telling us that the system does not work, then taking actions to make sure that it will not work, then telling us again, "See, we told you it didn't work." Over the past 25 years, this trend has been observable in area upon area of society. Perfectly healthy organisms, which may be in need of some consolidation or reorientation because of the normal effects of the passage of time, are instead undermined and then demonstrated to be faulty. These are the first steps towards replacing them with new structures that are intended to accomplish something completely different.

A short dithyramb will illustrate the point. Imagine that some private interests, political ideologues and civil servants wished to replace the comprehensive, universal, accessible Canadian medicare system with a two-tier structure which would gradually evolve in such a manner that the best services were in the private sector, as they are in Britain or, of course, the United States. Well, how would they go about it?

First, they would have to convince Canadians that their public system did not work. In order to accomplish this, they would have to be sure that the perfectly normal problems of age, from which the universal system — like any system — was suffering, were not addressed. Indeed they would have to work to accentuate those problems. How? Blunt, injudicious cutting would be a start. Better still, combine those cuts with the transfer of medical services to areas not properly integrated into medicare — to home care, for example. As services declined, waiting lists grew, patients suffered from isolation and poor service at home and medication bills piled up, well, the belief in universal medicare would be damaged. Suddenly the time would be ripe for a new "vision". And it would not be universal.

Of course, I am not suggesting that this is exactly what has happened. Nothing is ever so clear in reality. Rather, events unfold in a muddled manner over time. On the other hand, what has happened, what is happening, resembles this dithyramb. So whether those in a position to have some effect on events are guilty of intent or of incompetence is actually irrelevant. The citizenry increasingly distrust them because they are meant to be responsible for events.

Let me take this approach a little farther. Anyone who is an expert in a particular area should be very cautious about succumbing to the seductive fantasy that their innovative ideas will save the day. It might be better to take a more prudent approach and examine why it is they think something no longer works. There is a considerable difference, after all, between diagnosing a systemic problem that affects an entire organism, and identifying a symptomatic problem that requires not replacing the whole system, but rooting out the cause of the symptoms.

Although some observers today claim that the public health care system's current difficulties are actually systemic and argue for necessarily drastic change, I disagree. When I look at the five fundamental principles that were instituted and enshrined with medicare, I cannot discover anything wrong with them or, frankly, find anything that can be improved upon. I have yet to hear a convincing argument that today's issues cannot be addressed by medicare's original formula, and so require the amendment of its basic principles. Neither have I learned of anything to suggest that medicare's costs are spiraling out of control in a manner unforeseen in projections made at the time of its implementation. Cost figures which are, it is true, never entirely reliable, indicate that health care costs are about 20% under what Emmett Hall, one of the founders of medicare, thought they would be by this point.

CONVINCING US IT DOES NOT WORK

If the public health care system can still work as it was originally intended to, we have to wonder why recent governments seem so attached to the idea that it may not work at all. We also have to wonder why members of these governments, our duly elected representatives, seem to find it impossible to speak publicly about the current state of health care without lapsing into obfuscation or even outright mendaciousness. The Federal Minister of Trade, Sergio Marquis, part of a national government that until very recently had done its best to relinquish its historical role in health care, was quoted not long ago as saying, "People say health care is in danger; the reality is we are strengthening it." Similarly, in September of 1998, Quebec Premier Lucien Bouchard defended his government's policies by insisting that "we have the best system in the world."

The utterances of these two politicians are far from atypical: indeed, similarly improbable statements about medicare are made regularly in provincial capitals across Canada. But pronouncements of this kind typify a troubling reality for all Canadians. Although it is the job of our elected representatives to be the intellectual and practical voice of Canada's citizens — to understand the concerns of Canadians and develop policy that suitably addresses those concerns — the medicare debate is in fact handicapped by the attitudes and behaviour of politicians. To reassure us, they lie to us, and then treat us as idiots by insisting on things we all know are untrue. Not only does this prevent a reasonable debate from taking place, but it also creates a very unhealthy relationship between citizens and their elected representatives. The more politicians say everything is fine in the face of evidence to the contrary, the more the rest of us think there is something wrong with them. Quite correctly, we base our own estimation of the impact of events upon that which we observe and interpret around us. If the concerns and experiences of our families, friends, and communities seem to be consistently misunderstood and disregarded by the policy-makers whose decisions affect us, is it any wonder that sizeable numbers of Canadians feel alienated from their political elites?

The fear-mongering of our elected representatives has not helped matters either. Over the past few years, governments have steadily escalated their use of scare tactics in the health care debate. First, the public was told that fraud by patients was a major financial problem, if not the main problem, affecting the system. While there is undoubtedly a percentage of patients who do cheat — just as there are a percentage of chief executive officers who do not pay as much tax as they should, and a percentage of writers who do not write as good books as they should — a certain, marginal, amount of misuse is built into any system. There will always be a percentage of people who do not do what they are supposed to do. This is neither new nor unexpected. So why then was this minor factor suddenly presented as a central factor in decision making? The sensible answer is that fear-mongering is usually used to distract people from what is actually happening.

More recently, we were informed that it was doctors who were doing the cheating, and that it was once again a major problem. And, yes, some doctors are cheats, probably in percentages similar to the numbers of cheating patients and cheating CEOs, which is between .5% and 5%. It should be dealt with on a marginal basis. Instead, Ontario's health minister recently announced that the government intends to keep physicians honest by creating a report card system in which patients will report on what doctors are doing. The entire issue has been manipulated to create the impression among citizens-patients that they are being swindled by physicians. Enormous amounts of bureaucratic energy and public money will be wasted in this false control exercise, all in order to imbue the population with a sense of insecurity about the health care system and the people who make that system work. The stark reality is that this style of governance, based on state authority and public anxiety, uses a carrot-and-stick approach to avoid debate by dividing society through the creation of mistrust. Governance of this sort is also, interestingly enough, a quite natural and extreme form of modern managerial obsessions with control. I will come back to the role of the managerial system within public health care.

AN ANECDOTAL CRISIS

If we are to have a meaningful debate about health care, however, we need to be exact in the way we identify and acknowledge the real nature of the current crisis. Allan Rock, the current federal health minister, may say that he is not interested in "anecdotal evidence," but Canadians themselves are feeling the system's pulse in the stories they live and witness every day. Health care is not an abstraction. Nothing can be more exact, more existential, than the experience of patients. These experiences tell us a lot about where our system is failing us.

One example: An older man I know quite well was recently admitted to a large Toronto hospital for a specific problem. He found himself on a floor where there were one third of the nurses required to make the ward work. They were very good nurses, but they were so few that all they could do was look after basic needs and deal with emergencies in a reactive way. They had absolutely no time either to think about what was happening in that ward or to anticipate what might happen to those patients over the next period of time. Also, one had the sense that the doctors, while extremely competent, were nevertheless engaging in what I would call slightly heavy-handed care. The specialists were not really talking to each other about what effect each of their elements of care might have on an older man. They simply did not have the time to think about a soft-handed approach, a careful, integrated approach. They had to take clear, striking approaches to deal with a problem and move quickly on to something else.

The effect was that this older man went within three days from being a totally alert person to being a near-vegetable, rendered passive. In the process, as often happens with older people, he became incontinent, and we noticed after a period of time that he was lying around in his excrement. The nurses did not have time to change him as often as they should. Finally we asked why there were no diapers. The nurses, embarrassed, said that there was no money in the hospital budget for diapers. They told us quietly that we could buy diapers downstairs for $1.50 each. They were embarrassed about this because they are good nurses and they believe in medicare.

What I just described is not a universal medicare system but a two-tiered medical system. The people who have the money will hire a private nurse. They will go downstairs and buy the diapers. And the people who do not face the other prospect. And this in a hospital widely considered to be a model of "efficiency." I will come back to this concept. For the moment, it is enough to say that many of the problems I am discussing are the result of models of efficiency, and illustrate how misplaced the very utilitarian idea of efficiency is at the core of the medical system.

When he came out of the hospital, my friend went home. Indeed, there was the feeling that home care was the best way he could be treated. Everybody probably agrees that it is best for an older person to get out of the hospital system and home as quickly as possible. But to say that a hospital-centred medicare system is a problem and that a family, patient-centred system is what we need is nonsense unless home care is fully and utterly integrated into the medicare system. If not, what you are actually saying is that the medicare system cannot work. Why? Because the home care system, as it is currently set up, does not function as an integrated part of medicare. To abandon the hospital system in favour of the home care system, as currently organized, is, in fact, to privatize.

Public home care is so inadequate that it actually forces people to lie about what their situation is. For example, the ability to take a shower is one of the key factors deciding whether you will get publically funded home care. Some people can take showers but they cannot do the other things that make it possible to live at home. So, the patient has to be able to convince the authorities that they cannot take a shower in order to get help washing clothes or cleaning their house or whatever it is which will allow them to stay at home without living in filth. What is more, the tendency is to provide home care two or three times a week, meaning the elderly are to remain unwashed four or five days a week. The reality is that those who have the means use private home care. Again, it is a two-tier system. In addition, medications in the hospital system are part of medicare, while under home care, they must usually be paid for privately. Again, privatization and two-tier medicine. We are being treated as fools when we are told by our elected officials that there is nothing wrong with the medicare system. We are also being treated as fools by those who insist that medicare is a fundamentally flawed system which is failing as a result of its own weaknesses. In both cases we are being prevented from having a real debate about whether we want a two-tier system — about whether such a system is being denied and introduced at the same time in order to create a *fait accompli*. In spite of widespread and vehement disapproval for the idea, we continue to slip into a two-tier health care system.

THE ROOT OF THE PROBLEM

There is no denying that money is part of the problem, but it is also true that we are providing medicare for 20% less than Emmett Hall estimated we would be spending at this point. We are doing it for a great deal less than the Americans on a per capita basis. Therefore, there is room to spend more money. And no doubt we need more money in the system. Indeed, we are now told there will be more money. But I do not think that is the central problem. It is a result of the central problem. Tensions between the federal and provincial governments, which are an important part of the financial crisis, are a problem behind which everybody can hide. But, again, they are not the central problem.

POLICY NO LONGER DRIVEN BY IDEAS

Let me put foreword a very simple idea: Major public policies work when they are driven by ideas. As long as they are idea-driven, the most complex and almost impossible to imagine projects can work. That is the nature of public policy. If, and so long as, policies are idea-driven, they are on the offensive, and can work. The moment that a public policy is administration-driven, which is to say form-driven as opposed to content-driven, it doesn't work, no matter how hard you try to apply all of the administrative solutions being proposed.

We have seen many of these solutions over the past decade, and while the cutting and closings are presented as political solutions, they are really solutions that politicians have accepted from the administrative body, whether it is hospital boards or civil servants. These are administratively-driven reforms. And although we have done — again and again — what we have been asked to do, the effect has been that the medicare system works less and less well. That is because a public policy of this nature cannot work, the public good cannot work, when it is driven by administrative priorities. Once you start making those kinds of decisions, you slip deeper and deeper into a defensive position.

Form, management and efficiency

I mentioned the word efficiency. Administratively-driven structures are always obsessed by efficiency, in the private sector, in the public sector, in the arts, everywhere. But the concept of efficiency in western civilization is not what we have been led to believe. We have 2,500 hundred years of experience with different types of societies — democracies, dictatorships, benevolent dictatorships — and the fact is that, in western civilization, the concept of efficiency is at best a tertiary human quality. It is neither a great quality of capitalism nor of public service; it's just something you have to look after once you know what you want to do and where you want it to leave you. The promotion of efficiency to the senior level of policy making, has been one of the most disastrous innovations of our administratively-led medicare system.

The more "efficient" you make a medicare system, the less well — the less effectively — it will work. Note: I am not making an argument in favour of inefficiency. But allowing efficiency to drive the machine, while leaving the idea to follow hobbling behind, is extremely destructive. And it is a classic sign of a system which has lost its direction. People start claiming they will give us the direction by giving us efficiency. But you cannot get direction through efficiency. In fact you lose all possibility of direction. The more efficient and driven by administrative concerns, the less it works. Why? Because management is meaningless. Management contains absolutely no content, no meaning, no direction, no ideas. It is form, not content. And if we put managerial ideas in control, we have in fact induced the loss of direction in our system. It is a suicidal act. Management is necessary. You could even say management is essential. But then lots of elements are essential. Management only works effectively as a function or servant of policy.

How did management come to be given so much importance? We have never had so many managers. Hospitals and other institutions are more and more dominated by a managerial approach. Yet we have more and more managerial problems. And the more managerial problems there are, the more the managers talk about the need for leadership, by which they mean themselves. But of course management has nothing to do with leadership. Management is something which leaders require from people who work for them. The extent to which we have accepted the idea that managerial imperatives will give leadership is one of the key reasons it is now difficult to have a sensible discussion about medicare.

Management grew to this state of importance over about a hundred years as a kind of natural and necessary parasite of growing specialization among those who actually do something. The many groups of experts who do something in the medicare system disappear into their specializations and are split into narrower and narrower parallel specializations which have greater and greater difficulty talking to each other. Nothing actually holds the whole medicare system together except policy, or purpose, which is very hard to pursue without the participation of the experts. The only other thing remaining to hold it together, in the absence of the experts, is of course management. In a sense it is the abdication of the people who represent "content" which makes inevitable the rise to power of those who are merely managers of form. This is not an attack on managers, but an attack on the role we have given to management.

Policy and content are dependent on the citizens and on elected officials but, in the long run, they are dependent on the experts. By that I do not mean the experts as an expert interest group, but the experts in their role as expert citizens. The abdication of the expert from that role has become a dangerous flaw in the western democratic system. When experts abandon policy they create a vacuum which management fills. Doctors, especially, abandon policy because they have been told that rising levels of complexity and specialization mean that they must concentrate on their area and that nobody outside of their area is going to understand what they are talking about. In other words they abandon it because they accept the rise of what I call corporatism. They accept that the way society will run is not through the legitimacy of citizens acting together and bringing their expertise to the public table. Instead, they accept that society works as thousands and thousands of interest groups, each functioning on the inside and leaving it to someone else — the managers — to pull it all together.

Corporatism is precisely the system proposed by Benito Mussolini in the 1920s and '30s. It is precisely that system which we have now adopted in a sort of cleaned up professional modern form without actually recognizing it as the system we went to war to fight against a half century ago.

Interest mediation

What we are left with is an interest-based, expert-based society where relationships between the interests, between the specialized groups, between the corporations, are based on what they now call interest mediation; the liver specialist mediates with the brain surgeon, and health care mediates with the banking sector; compromises are made not with a larger idea in mind, but on the basis of interest and self-interest. This is the basic concept of corporatism, whether it is applied to medicine, business or public interest, and it does not actually work because society is not based on a compromise between two competing interests.

Hospital-based or disease-based medicine provides a concrete place in which that interest mediation can take place. A health-based or citizen-based, that is patient-based approach to health care cannot be dealt with on the basis of interest mediation, of corporatism. In other words we have fallen increasingly into the Conradian trap described when a character said of Lord Jim: "Strictly speaking the question is not how to get cured but how to live." We have gone in exactly the opposite direction.

The kind of cuts that have been made in the last few years accentuate this process, because they drive the system to concentrate on the highest intensity of care. If we have so little time and money, and so many people with such narrow expertise, that we are not able to think, we will increasingly fall into providing high intensity care and avoid low intensity care which involves thinking about the shape of society.

As managerial systems grow, they assert their methods. "Quality assurance" is one such method, a classic managerial phrase that means absolutely nothing. Quality of what? It has nothing to do with quality in terms which a 19th century doctor or a humanist doctor of the 20th century would understand. The phrase reflects an obsession with measuring which comes when efficiency becomes a goal in and of itself. So much time is spent processing data and statistics on what we are doing that there is no time to think about the realities of society —and thus of patients — and even less to think about what we could be doing. We become stuck in a present that cuts out both past and future and so succumb to a kind of utilitarian inevitability.

You could say that we have become obsessed by data over information. Or that we have become so obsessed by narrow, exclusive, apparently controllable forms of data that we have excluded the wider, inclusive sort. In other words, that we have created narrow, data-based artificial realities as a way of denying reality itself. Reality? That larger place with a past, a present and a future and a lateral complexity of uncontrollable factors.

REINTEGRATING KNOWLEDGE, THOUGHT AND ACTION IN PATIENT-CENTRED HEALTH CARE

A patient-centred approach to health care requires openness and cooperation on a non-interested basis among experts, citizens and governments. It requires transparency, public involvement, debate.

Under a corporatist technocracy the disease-based approach is preferred because it is much more controllable. Everything is locked up among the experts who are themselves locked up underneath the managerial system. In managerial terms, success is, first and foremost, about control.

We have an enormous need for an integrated approach. We need information about our population, about what people want and what they are experiencing, and about where they are headed. We need to understand how they live and can live. For example, sending people home to "home care" when there is no family at home or within miles is not sending them home. It is sending them to solitary confinement. We need to think about that information and, out of those thoughts, develop policies.

More than anything, we need to reconnect knowledge, thought and action as three steps which are both integrated and integral to one another. At present, they are hopelessly disconnected. The policies we are getting have nothing to do with the information which has become available. Information about what is happening in society is not particularly welcomed in a management-driven system because it suggests that there is something other than a managerial imperative at work, that people may also recognize a social imperative and want to see it represented in the health care system. Management fears thought because thought is a form of disorder. And it fears the integration of thought and action even more. Why? Because it suggests an inability to control things. Therefore, management is afraid to acknowledge information which suggests that things cannot be easily controlled.

The overwhelming sense of passivity and frustration among doctors, nurses and other experts in the health care field comes, I believe, from being locked up in corporations. Frustration stems from an unwillingness to accept passivity, to accept that they are unable to affect public policy. Nevertheless, there is a sense of inevitability, of not being able to choose directions. It suddenly seems impossible to choose among three directions because it is impossible to admit that there could be three valid directions. It seems equally impossible to look at the data collected and make decisions accordingly. For example, it seems there is an enormous amount of data indicating that smaller hospitals work best for many kinds of care. And yet the policies now in place are leading to larger and larger hospitals. Without proper public debate about why the data says one thing and the policies are doing another thing, we are going in the direction of the managerial imperative, not in the direction of the information. Indeed, there is not even a debate questioning why these issues are not being debated.

The inability to digest and make use of the information we have is an example of what happens when people feel a great sense of passivity and frustration, and when our structures are management driven. Doctor Oliveri's battle in the context of the Hospital for Sick Children over what is the proper ethical approach toward research, in particular privately-funded research, is a case in point. It is not simply about private sector influence on research. Beyond that it is about whether knowledge brings power, which is to say control, or whether knowledge brings communication and debate. In a healthy health care system, knowledge brings communication and debate. The company's representative was quoted as saying, "This is not a matter of public debate." In other words, they were terrified by the idea that their information would get out and be spoken about by non-experts who were not locked up and divided into their various public and private and professional corporations.

The Nobel prize winning scientist, John Polanyi made the following, I think very wise, comment on the Oliveri case: "What we are seeing here is not a problem particular to medical science but a more general one stemming from the ever increasing commercialization, at the university, of research. The purpose of research is to uncover the truth and if this is to stand a chance of succeeding, it must be pursued openly, so that little by little the truth can be winnowed out in debate. That debate must be free, and be seen to be free from commercial and political influence." What he is commenting on and what I am commenting on is not simply a problem with university research, but a much more general problem that affects private as well as public sectors, industry as well as academia. We must not forget that the private sector is also managerially-driven and suffers to an equal if not greater extent from the negative consequences of corporatism described above.

It is worth remembering that, in Canada, we pay for the education of the experts, we pay for the places in which they perform their functions, and we do that because we expect the experts to be our voice, our experts. Not the system's experts, but our experts. That apart from saving our lives, for which we are extremely grateful on a daily basis, we expect them to tell us how the system is working and to talk to us, openly, about the various ways in which they think it could be made to work better. At present, they are unable to play that role, both because they have increasingly been excluded from the debate, and because they have found it more difficult to get into the debate in a disinterested manner that focuses on the public good.

It has become very difficult not only to have any public debate, but to have any kind of integrated thinking in public. Let me give you an example of the effect that this has on public policy. Health Canada is now holding hearings around the country about renewing the federal health protection legislation, for which they prepared a document called "Shared Responsibility, Shared Visions." In it, Health Canada invites "partners and other stakeholders to join in this discussion." There is no suggestion anywhere in the document that health care is something that actually belongs to the citizens. Rather, it belongs to the stakeholders. The whole notion of stakeholders is based on a corporatist dictate that the only time citizens can claim a seat at the table is when they are interested parties. Not by virtue of being a disinterested citizen, but by virtue of being an interested party engaged in interest mediation. The word stakeholder is so omnipresent throughout this document that as I read it I could not help thinking that universal medicare is dying because it has a stakeholder through the heart. At every level, the debate has been reduced to deciding what roles various stakeholders should play. At this table, the citizen is reduced to a consumer.

Our experts are increasingly prisoners of their own system. This prevents them from seeing themselves as citizens, even though they know they are citizens. They have great difficulty distancing themselves from the concept of self-interest, which is supposed to drive them, and which is rewarded in this society. Too often we see doctors try to intervene in a helpful way only to end up adopting a stance that sends exactly the wrong message to the public — a corporatist self-interested message. That is what happens in a society like this. It becomes very difficult for any of us, writers, doctors, politicians, to find our way into the public debate in a helpful manner. The system does not reward that kind of participation, so we are constantly urged to deform the way we think into something which would make sense in a corporatist society. I am convinced that doctors are primarily concerned with the public interest, but they have yet to find a way into the debate as a voice for the public interest, as opposed to the corporation.

There is a great need, at the moment, for an aggressive change in self-perception among all of us who are involved in health care. I say "us" because I mean the citizen as responsible individual, as patient and as expert. We face the challenge of building the role of the public good back into the system. Corporations create the illusion that people inside the corporations are protected by them, and that is what produces the sense that knowledge is about control. Protection itself is about control. The reality, especially in medicine, is that transparency is the only thing that makes sense and works well.

In the midst of all of this, I think we forget the astonishingly important role that health care experts have played in the creation, throughout the western world, of democracy, indeed, of the kind of society we live in. I think doctors themselves forget, when they are looking for models which might guide them toward intervention in the system, that to a very great extent, the shape of this country was determined by a series of remarkable doctors such as the great Dr. Baldwin from Toronto, father of Robert Baldwin. Among other things, he set up perhaps the first free public medicine hospital in Canada. He was the first major public figure to show that medicine could be other than an interest-based system. And he was the "godfather" of the democratic reforms of the 1830s and '40s. Dr. Wolfred Nelson, military leader of the Patriots in 1837, was later the first popularly elected mayor of Montreal and the first doctor to carry out an operation under anaesthetic in Canada. Nova Scotia's Dr. Charles Tupper was the father of public education, of universal male suffrage, not to mention of confederation. Doctors have always been central to Canadian society, just as the health care system has always been central to Canadians' idea of themselves.

In a way, this country was created through a series of great leaps, in which we applied a specific, but extremely important idea in a practical manner to the running of the public good. I call these great leaps in practical metaphysics. The application of each of these has become a central illustration of how people of that era thought their society should work. And so, from that practical centre, a whole series of other ideas and policies would reverberate into place and shape our society. Medicare was one of those great leaps. When we put it in place it was clear what kind of society we wanted. And as a result a whole series of other policies came into being, dealing with other issues but reflecting the principles, the ethics, the public standards of medicare.

Let me sum up the points I have made about where health care now stands in Canada:

First, medicare can only work if it is driven by ideas, by policy.

Second, our growing dependency on managers is killing medicare, not openly, but behind a pervasive rhetoric that claims to be saving it through such utilitarian dogmas as "efficiency" at the expense of the practical application of ideas which would result in such concepts as "effectiveness."

Third, the refusal of publicly elected figures to speak out frankly and honestly about what is happening to medicare is actually blocking useful public debate and is therefore doing a great deal of damage. Their fear of admitting what is happening is facilitating that decline.

Fourth, medical experts have largely accepted that health care must be organized according to corporatist structures. As a result they are denying to society their help in asserting the sort of ideas which could produce a new generation of universal medicare.

Fifth, the result of the failure of both the political and the expert elites to play their roles has been that we have slipped into a two-tier health care system without any public debate over whether citizens wished to abandon the universal system. Worse still, our elites continue to talk as if we still have a universal system. They, and therefore we, condemn ourselves to live a lie.

Sixth, this situation is made worse by the natural managerial tendency to discourage and punish integrated thinking and to create levels of distrust among citizens separated into interest groups.

Seventh, the abstract, control-oriented approach typical of a management-dominated corporatist system leads to the simple denial of such obvious problems as the shortage of nurses and the destructive delisting of certain services.

Eighth, there is a great need for the public sector to collect data on a patient-centred approach to health care and, having collected it, to accept the sequential relationship between information, thought and policy, something that has been almost totally denied for a decade. The relationship between these three elements are what ties ideas of the public good to the reality of the public good. Why? Because they cut across the artificial, abstract, top-down and interest-driven divisions of corporatism. In accepting corporatist structures, medical experts have largely denied their real strengths and their ability to play a central role in finding new directions. Only by walking away from that acceptance of corporatism as the determining model in society can doctors and other experts play their proper role in changing the direction of health care. I believe they can do this, and frankly we do not stand a chance without them.

And finally, ninth, as a first step in the direction of a patient-centred approach to health care, I believe, as do many others (we call ourselves citizens), we must move quickly to establish a full home care system that is completely integrated — financially, administratively, and expertly integrated — into the medicare system. That obviously must include medication costs. Home care is a perfect illustration or adaptation of three of the five principles of the Canada Health Act: comprehensiveness, universality and accessibility. The idea of home care fits into the original definition of medicare. There may be enormous political problems in establishing such a system, but all important developments are politically problematic in Canada; that is the nature of our country. And frankly, to cut back on the hospital system, which is integrated into medicare, while throwing responsibility onto a home care system which is not, is a dangerous — and more precisely, a dishonest — way to introduce a two-tier health care system without seeking any public approval.

In order to reestablish such basic principles as comprehensiveness, universality and accessibility through a properly integrated home care system, we must ensure that our intent, the idea we want to bring about, is publicly stated and debated. There is nothing to be gained by holding back from putting that "content" directly on the table. There is nothing to be gained by political figures hedging on it because they are afraid that somebody is going to ask them for money. We need to have the debate about purpose. Then we can have the debate about money. Then we can have the political debate. First we deal with the idea, then we move to the utilitarian problem of money, then we move to the pure politics. If we decide that we care, and choose the direction we want to go in, then we will find a way to make it happen.

CHAPTER 2

Clinical Considerations in Health Policy

The Impact of Health Policy on Clinical Decisions and the Doctor-Patient Relationship

Dr. Richard Cruess and Dr. Sylvia Cruess

Before addressing the impact of health policy on clinical practice, we will begin by briefly stating our views on the issues we plan to neglect; issues that are the mainstay of current debates on the future of clinical practice. For one, we do not intend to discuss the idea of a privatized parallel sector in the health care system. We are firmly committed to a single standard of care and do not consider it possible to achieve this objective in the presence of a parallel private sector open only to those who can afford it. We also believe, however, that it is morally wrong and politically impossible in the long run to ban a private sector unless the public system is funded and structured in ways that will meet society's needs and satisfy public expectations. In this regard, we believe (as do the vast majority of Canadians) that our health care system is presently underfunded due to a series of decisions made by all levels of government. We did not believe this five years ago.

What we are witnessing in Canada is democracy at work, and it has been interesting. Health and health care are now firmly situated in the political arena where they are heavily influenced by political forces. Public opinion on the adequacy of health care funding reflects subjective feelings as much as it does scientific and economic analysis, and any level of funding that makes clinical care inconvenient and inadequate will not be acceptable for long. Ultimately, public expectations will do more to drive political agendas than any set of outcome measurements, and many forces, including the advice of the medical profession, will inform public perception on this matter. If the public continues to believe that funding is insufficient, there will be ongoing pressure to either increase funding or to establish a private sector.

Having said that, let us assume money will be put back into health care in Canada because of present and future public pressure; that the federal and provincial governments will restore at least some of the funding removed from the system. This will solve some of the present difficulties concerning both access and quality and may even ease some of the current stresses upon the doctor-patient relationship. It is no secret that many physicians feel they cannot provide optimum care with the resources available. However, restoration of funding will not transform our health care system into one in which there is an easy synergy between policy making and practice. For that to happen we must reestablish a reasonable working relationship between the medical profession and the policy-makers, and it is this topic that we wish to address.

A REASONABLE WORKING RELATIONSHIP

In modern times there has been an implicit agreement between society and its professions. This agreement evolved without formal structure until the late 19th century, became firmly fixed in the 20th century, and began to be criticized after the Second World War. These criticisms had an impact on public policy at a time when the professions were firmly entrenched and resistant to any change that would alter their status. The bureaucracies of professional associations were well-established, conservative and powerful. Throughout the western world, medicine consistently failed to understand the details of its bargain with the societies it was meant to serve.

When Canada and the United Kingdom made the political decision to establish universal health care, for example, the medical profession initially chose to resist rather than collaborate. Physicians did not understand that they were subject to political control through the democratic process. The profession failed to comprehend that professional status is not an inherent right but, rather, something granted by society with the expectation that professionals would meet certain obligations in return. In turn, the failure in the United States to reach any firm consensus on how to organize the delivery of health care, a failure in no small part attributable to the American Medical Association's intense lobbying efforts, has led to a market-driven system in that country which appears to please very few.

In examining the evolution of the health care professions and their relationship to society, it is easy to identify heroes and villains. What one tends to forget is that access to care, quality of care, and the doctor-patient relationship are largely influenced by practitioners who are neither heroic nor villainous. They are simply health care providers, doing their best to function within a constantly changing system over which they feel they have little control. Now, for the first time in many years, there is an opportunity to re-establish trust and communication between medicine and society and make things better. But before looking into the future, it is important to continue looking at the impact of past policies to put our present situation in a historical context.

THE IMPACT OF PAST POLICIES

There are some services which societies have always required, such as the care of the sick, the adjudication of disputes, and the meeting of spiritual needs. As these functions become increasingly complex, more and more expertise is required to fulfill them, and their organization grows ever more difficult. Since the 19th century, society has used the evolving concept of the profession as a means of organizing the delivery of these services, including health care. Contemporary physicians are expected to simultaneously occupy two major roles, those of healer and professional, which are inextricably linked in the minds of the public and the medical profession itself. The roles share much common ground, but are drawn from different traditions and entail different sets of obligations, neither of which can be ignored without altering the relationship between medicine and society. However, these dual roles have become increasingly confused in the analysis of both societal and professional expectations; the rich literature on professionalism found in sociology and ethics, for example, most often discusses them together. This is unfortunate, as anecdotal evidence indicates that neither society nor physicians currently have a clear understanding of the interaction of the two roles. We in turn suggest that they be understood and utilized separately for very sound operational reasons.

THE PHYSICIAN AS HEALER AND PROFESSIONAL

The tradition of the physician healer in western society dates back to Hippocrates and is known and cherished by medical practitioners everywhere. The Hippocratic Oath forms the cornerstone of the medical profession's morality and self-image, and is treated with such respect that the oath is an important shared element of western culture. Even today, both physicians and patients probably have a fairly accurate conception of the role of the healer.

The origins of professionalism, on the other hand, are more recent and have evolved differently in different countries. In the English-speaking world, the relative historical weakness of the state and the traditions already existing in the guilds and universities of England saw the professions evolve into independent and self-regulating bodies. As the Industrial Revolution provided society with the means to purchase health care, science made it worth buying. In order to organize what had become a chaotic field of endeavour, laws were then passed that created mandates for independent professional bodies and established licensure. For the first time, these legal measures granted medicine a broad monopoly over health care along with both individual and collective autonomy. However — and this is extremely important — this was done with the clear understanding that in return, medicine would concern itself with the health problems of the society it served and would place the welfare of that society above its own. From the beginning, the autonomy granted to the profession entailed clearly defined obligations, yet many of these obligations had and still have only a remote connection to the role of physician as healer. One can make the point that we in medicine have not failed as much as healers as we have as professionals.

Defining professionalism

It is axiomatic that the role of the healer depends on professional status and that healing is jeopardized by unprofessional behaviour. It is surprising, then, that most professionals do not fully understand professionalism or its obligations. The *Oxford English Dictionary* defines a profession as "the occupation which one professes to be skilled in and to follow: a) a vocation in which a professed knowledge of some department of learning or science is used in application to the affairs of others or in the practice of an art founded upon it; b) in a wider sense, any calling or occupation by which a person habitually earns his or her living."[1] The word "profess" is important. For a physician, the Hippocratic Oath represents a public profession of commitment which cannot be ignored. However, for those of us working in the Anglo-American tradition, this dictionary definition does not include important characteristics of what we understand a profession to be.

The core of every profession contains two major elements: possession of a specialized body of knowledge and a commitment to service. From these core values follow all others. Self-regulation is granted to those who have specialized knowledge because that knowledge is not really available to society, and it is felt that the quality of service will be assured by the process of self-regulation. Autonomy is given on the understanding that professionals will devote themselves to serving others rather than themselves. In the case of medicine, the profession has agreed upon values and a code of ethics so that the professional role may support that of the healer. All professions must be intrinsically moral: they act for the benefit of society and the justification for their monopoly rests on their conduct. Accordingly, professionalism is an ideal which must be pursued in practice by all professionals, though it is understood that as fallible human beings we sometimes fall short of our ideals. Thus, unreasonable objectives are not set.

Much of the maintenance of the professions has been assigned to licensing bodies and professional associations whose mandates in this country are derived from the Canadian Parliament or provincial legislatures. The setting and maintenance of standards, self-regulation, the development of codes of ethics, and informing the public and legislative authorities are all important parts of these mandates. Support of these organizations and their activities becomes a professional obligation.

Changing views of medicine

At this point, it is useful to review the body of literature on the professions. A review is not just an academic exercise. The views in the literature both reflect and shape public opinion, and have had a significant effect on the formation of public policy. The literature pertaining to the theory of professions and to professional behaviour can be categorized in different ways, but for our purposes it is most useful to look at its evolution chronologically. The early literature, up to just after the Second World War, was largely descriptive of and favourable to the concept of professionalism. It includes works by many social scientists who helped to define present-day society: Weber, Durkheim, Beatrice and Sydney Webb, Tawney, Flexner, Brandeis, Saunders, and Parsons all endorsed the concept of professionalism because they believed that professionals would be altruistic. Even when they identified the inherent tension between altruism and self-interest, these thinkers hypothesized that it was in the best interest of the professional to be altruistic and that professionals therefore would be. This was at a time when authority was respected, and the professions were largely responsible for the shape of health care systems. They were regarded as impartial experts, even if evidence sometimes indicated otherwise.

In the 1960s and '70s, criticism of western society became more frequent and generalized, and the professions did not escape notice. Elliot Freidson was the first, and in many ways, the most influential critic of contemporary medicine. Freidson assembled a large and consistent body of learning to stress that medicine had used its control over its knowledge base to gain a dominant position in society and within the health care field. He also noted the inherent conflict between altruism and self-interest, and pointed out medicine's spectacular failure to self-regulate. Medical professionals had collectively put their own welfare above that of the society their profession was meant to serve.

Other critics including McKinley, Larsen, Haug, Johnson, and Starr, contributed powerful arguments. They commented on the closed nature of the professions, predicted that medicine would lose much of its status because of changes in modern society, and anticipated many of the economically driven changes now seen in the United States, described as the "proletarianization of medicine." Medicine was characterized as being involved in a "collective mobility project" in which it sought to improve its position in society with little or no thought for the public good.[2] It was felt that the medical profession organized itself in order to gain a monopoly over a service, and controlled its market in order to create a demand for service. The work of these critics all stressed the self-serving power of a professional elite and its impact on social policy. Collectively, this work had an enormous influence on those who were making public policy, and medicine lost much of its ability to alter policy. It was not trusted.

The literature of the past 15 years shows a subtle change that we will venture to explain before describing. Up until the Second World War, medicine effectively controlled its market. It controlled entry into the workplace, the conditions of employment, methods and amount of payment, and the structure of the health care system. Starting with the development of commercial insurance and then various national health schemes, including those in the United States, control of the marketplace had shifted by the 1990s, a process beautifully documented in Elliot Krause's *Death of the Guilds*.[3] The health care system has become almost completely dominated by either the state or capitalism, and the professions have thus lost power, a situation well understood by the public. Rudolf Klein, a wonderfully wise sociologist in Britain, once recommended that the state leave sufficient control over health care to the medical profession so the profession could share in the blame for problems.[4] This has not occurred, and in the public eye it is now the state, or in the United States, the state and marketplace, which are held responsible for flaws in the health care system.[5]

Perhaps as a result, recent literature is kinder both to the medical profession and to the concept of professionalism. In Freidson's latest book, *Professionalism Reborn*, he examines different means of organizing medical services and concludes that professionalism, despite its defects, remains the least unattractive method of organization.[6] Other authors, besides ourselves, agree with Freidson's conclusions but stress that professionalism, as such, must be clearly understood by both society and physicians. It must be a professionalism in which service is once again paramount. Freidson, who has always been sympathetic to individual physicians while criticizing the profession's collective behaviour, is optimistic. Krause, conversely, is not. Here it is worth quoting from the last paragraph of his *Death of the Guilds*, which summarizes what may well be the views of many contemporary professionals and health care consumers:

> The result for the average patient may well be poorer quality care by an even more overburdened staff. Perhaps consumers no longer feel that they can influence the state on their behalf or even reach the politicians who are primarily responding to capitalist interests and not their own. Perhaps this too is but a phase. My guess is that it is not, and that the processes at work here represent a great threat to the health and welfare of us all. The question remains: What can be done to resist what appears to be an irresistible tide?[7]

THE STATE OF THE PROFESSION: THREE REASONS FOR OPTIMISM

Having thought long and hard about these issues, we believe that if the medical profession responds appropriately, it can once again affect policy decisions and make substantial improvements in areas like access to care and quality of care. There are three major reasons for our optimism. The first relates to faith in the democratic process and its relationship with organized medicine, and is reinforced by medicine's contemporary acceptance of its deferential role to the democratic process and the loss of marketplace control this entails. The state now controls physician numbers, levels of remuneration and, in some instances, methods of remuneration. It also administers the structure of the system within which physicians work, but has left medicine's value system and the setting, maintenance and enforcement of standards to the profession, while requiring a more open and transparent system. Values remain the concern of the profession, while financial and administrative matters are largely controlled by others, which may at least allow medicine to try to return to its original ideals.

The second reason to be optimistic springs from the first. As the medical profession no longer controls the health care system, its counsel on health care is now less self-interested and more respectable, and its role as expert has been re-established. Unlike Brint, we believe that the social trusteeship model of professionalism is compatible with the expert model.[8] This is new and offers real opportunities if professional associations recognize them. We do see some evidence of this recognition; in the last two years the Canadian Medical Association has rejected a privatized system and has been quite effective in addressing the issue of funding without mentioning physician remuneration.

There is a third cause for optimism, one which is probably the most significant. Society's need for and dependence on the healer is very great. Because of this, we believe that trends observed in other professions will continue to be somewhat blunted in medicine. While there has been a change in the status and power of the medical profession, it has nonetheless retained much of the healer's mystique in the public's eye. The latest Harris Poll in the United States places medicine at the top of a list of prestigious occupations, with 61% of the American public believing that physicians enjoy "very great prestige," a percentage that has increased by 11% since 1992. The public remains medicine's greatest ally and wants a trusting relationship with the profession. The past few decades had seen a deterioration of the relationship because physicians were perceived as being primarily interested in increasing their own incomes and power. Paradoxically, with the loss of the profession's power base and ability to control its own market, there now appears to be an opportunity to rebuild trust. Indeed, it is clear that the public wants physicians to make major decisions regarding its health, rather than those representing either the state or the marketplace. For this to occur, however, the public must be able to regard physicians and their associations as consistently acting in a self-disinterested fashion.

It is not enough to offer an analysis of how we have arrived where we are, and then simply express optimism or pessimism. There is a distinct need to develop guidelines for future action. In order to have an opportunity to improve the current system, all health care professions, including medicine, must return to their core values, properly analyze their contract with society, and carry out responsibilities formulated in terms of service to society. The healer must serve the individual patient first and society second, and professional associations and licensing bodies must support the healer and serve society.

SOME SPECIFIC POINTS

1. The primacy of the role of healer must be recognized. As stated earlier, we believe that medicine's failures in this area have been noted, and that there have been substantial efforts mounted in order to correct them. Codes of ethics are more effective and appropriate than they were and are more widely publicized; one hopes that they have more influence on physician behaviour. Discipline within the profession is becoming more rigorous within a more open system. It is crucial that these efforts continue and that every physician support them.

2. Physicians must reassert their commitment to individual patients: a commitment that must be seen by patients as taking precedence over any obligation to society as a whole. If the patient feels that the physician is making decisions while prioritizing what has been called distributive justice, all basis for trust in that physician will be jeopardized. We believe that understanding this is of great importance to the physician, to the medical profession, and especially to policy-makers. The healer and the advocate for the individual patient cannot be separated.

3. Professional associations have two major functions. They have a mandated duty to set and maintain standards, to discipline uneth-

ical and unprofessional conduct, and to concern themselves with societal problems. However, they are also expected to represent their members and fulfill a union function, as do respected organizations such as the British Medical Association and the Fédération des médecins spécialistes du Québec, both of which are legal unions. Nevertheless, when an association is perceived by the public as putting the welfare of its members first, it seriously compromises its ability to influence public policy, even when its recommendations are judicious and in the best interests of society. In many jurisdictions there is a legal separation of these functions, but all medical associations and licensing bodies can lose their credibility as advocates for positive change in the health care system if they are felt to be concerned mainly with serving their own members. Therefore, medicine must evolve towards a system in which the two functions become more clearly separated than they are now: if this is not possible, the formation of some type of Canadian Health Council to fulfill the advocacy role may be required. In any event, history demonstrates that a trusted medical association can use its expertise in the best interests of society and be a force for good.

4. Physicians must support their professional associations. The legal mandates of these associations clearly give them a role in shaping important institutions and serving society, and the credibility of the association is heavily dependent upon participation by its members. If a physician is unhappy with the direction of an association, there is an obligation to attempt to change that direction rather than withdrawing.

5. All physicians must be aware of the extent of their professional obligations, a situation which does not now exist. They must know and understand the national and regional laws and regulations, fully understand the codes of professional behaviour designed to govern their conduct, and participate in a more effective and transparent process of self-regulation in order to achieve accountability. They must also be involved in health issues pertaining to

societal problems such as access to health care services and resource allocation, and be fully accountable for all decisions taken. This responsibility requires that physicians base their practice on sound evidence and maintain competence throughout their careers.

At the same time, there are obligations which require special emphasis in today's world. The centrality of our knowledge base means that each of us shares an obligation to expand and ensure its integrity; science must be supported and scientific fraud addressed. Although the intrusion of both the state and the marketplace has significantly affected the autonomy of medical practitioners, every physician is obliged to refuse to practice in a situation where they are not free to make independent decisions about the best care for patients. Finally, all physicians must be governed by professional standards, whether employed as private practitioners, employees of hospitals, universities, governments or corporations, or as managers, administrators or those filling multiple roles.

In conclusion

As we have written elsewhere,[9] these measures will require educational campaigns aimed at students, trainees, practicing physicians and associations, as well as the general public. These recommendations are made on the assumption that our health care system has ceased to function properly in part because professionals failed to meet many of their obligations. If physicians fulfill their roles as both healers and professionals, their enhanced credibility can lead to better policy decisions that will have a positive impact on access to and quality of care, as well as the doctor-patient relationship.

Lastly, we want to reemphasize the importance of a historical perspective. The last 50 years have seen the deconstruction of the structures and institutions put into place in the 19th century and strengthened in the first half of the 20th century. Much of that social order is gone for good. Because of their part in that order, medical professionals and the concept of service were placed under intense pressure, and the ability of even the most well-meaning professional to influence the course of events was diminished. We believe that the medical profession now finds itself in a different situation. For the first time in many decades, there is a confluence between what the public wants and what the profession wishes. If individual practitioners and their professional institutions fully understand both their redefined contract with society and its resultant obligations and act vigorously to fulfill these obligations, a better health care system should result.

We end by agreeing with Sullivan, who stressed the importance of integrity to the professions, believing that neither economic incentives, technology, or bureaucratic control could replace the inner commitment evoked by professionalism.[10]

End notes

1. *Oxford English Dictionary*, 2nd ed. Oxford, U.K: Clarendon Press,. 1989.
2. McKinley, J.B. "Toward proletarianization of physicians." In Deber, E., ed. *Professionals as Workers: Mental Labour in Advanced Capitalism*. Boston, MA: G.K. Hall, 1982. pp. 37-62.
3. Krause, E. *Death of the Guilds: Professions, States and the Advance of Capitalism, 1930 to the Present.* New Haven, CT: Yale University Press, 1996.
4. Klein, R. "National variations in international trends." in Hafferty, F.W. and McKinlay, J.B. *The Changing Medical Profession: An International Perspective.* New York: Oxford University Press, 1993. pp. 202-209.
5. Cruess, R.L. and Cruess, S.R. "Teaching medicine as a profession in the service of healing." *Academic Medicine* 72, 1997. pp. 941-952.
6. Freidson, R. *Professionalism Reborn.* Chicago, Ill: University of Chicago Press, 1994.
7. Op. cit. page 286.
8. Brint, S. *In an Age of Experts: The Changing Role of Professionals in Politics and Public Life.* Princeton, NJ: Princeton University Press, 1994.
9. Cruess and Cruess, as above.
10. Sullivan, W. *Work and Integrity: The Crisis and Promise of Professionalism in America.* New York: Harper Collins, 1995.

Creating a Sound Clinical Basis for Health Policy: Three Views

Bringing the Patient on Board

Pat Kelly

Canada's health care system is currently experiencing many problems. Despite the $12.5 billion in federal funds spent annually on medicare, the standard of care is not acceptable to many Canadians, and the public is angry and frustrated that constant tensions between different levels of government, institutions, and health professionals are affecting care and patients' relationships with their physicians. The gulf that now exists between patients and practitioners, payers and politicians reflects the public's deepening lack of confidence in the medicare system; a crisis of confidence that mirrors an intense personal frustration among many Canadians. It is a sense of frustration that comes from dealing with a health care system that seems to have lost touch with its essential mission to serve the needs of sick people.

Support for a publicly funded single-payer health care system has never been granted unequivocally by Canadians. Instead, it has always been given in exchange for timely and universal access to the highest possible quality of care. Although public opinion surveys have consistently found that health care users are satisfied with the quality of technical care they receive, there is an increasing perception of serious shortcomings in the standard of care offered. Trust in the health care system has declined dramatically, and major changes are necessary if the system is to regain the confidence of Canadians. Public opinion surveys across Canada have repeatedly shown that Canadians prioritize the improvement and increased funding of health care above all of government's other responsibilities, including education, employment, and culture.

A failure to respond to declining public confidence will have far reaching consequences for health care. After all, it is high public esteem that has always sustained the considerable investment and substantial privileges granted to the health care system and its providers. The downward trend in public confidence parallels the federal government's declining share of public expenditures, from 42% in 1978, to the current low of 29%. At the same time, while the case has been made that the public remains the health professional's greatest ally, the relationship between doctors and patients has also deteriorated. Time is now so limited in many medical encounters that the human relationship between caregiver and patient has suffered, and Canadians, like their American counterparts, are turning to other types of healers for the consultation, care, and comforting they need.

In this manner, a 1993 Health Canada survey of cancer survivors reported that more than a third of respondents used some form of alternative therapy. In the same year, a U.S. study by David Eisinger, published in the *New England Journal of Medicine*, estimated that one out of every three Americans used unconventional treatments. The study indicated that one in four medical patients used alternative therapies, and that seven out of ten did not discuss the use of these therapies with their physician. Expenditures associated with the use of these therapies amounted to approximately $13.7 billion U.S., three quarters of it paid out of pocket.

One explanation for the large-scale use of unproven alternative therapies by otherwise savvy consumers is that patients often resort to healers because the latter introduce a note of caring and validation into treatment in ways that contemporary physicians do not. To quote Robert Buckman's book *Magic or Medicine*: "Patients go to healers, whether the treatments work or not, because it is comforting and because it is the socially valid thing to do." Diseases need medicine, but human beings who suffer will always need a touch of magic. While this trend may be part of a growing cynicism in North American society about the medical profession, it is rooted in changes in patients' experiences of care that emerged with the evolution of modern medicine over the last fifty years. In their work at the Picker Institute, Thomas Moloney and Barbara Paul identified four major changes that alienated patients from the medical profession. In their view, the increasing specialization in the training of medical practitioners, explosive development of information technologies, and increased burden of cost for patients all combined with shifting generational values to undermine North Americans' traditional faith in the medical system.

Moloney and Paul refer to this shift as "the shattering of the Osler tradition," after the great Victorian medical clinician who did so much to determine the course of 20th century medicine in North America. Even as recently as the 1940s, medical practice in this country was still very much in the tradition of the Osler Master Clinician. Osler-style practice relied on the establishment of a personal relationship based on trust and confidence between physician and patient. That relationship was an explicit part of the therapeutic process, and a physician would comfort patients, give them confidence in their own ability to do well, and share personal feelings as a matter of course. It is no coincidence that patients attribute these same qualities of compassion and warmth, openness, knowledge and humour to their alternative practitioners. Conversely, as physicians have specialized, the art of ministering to the whole patient has gradually faded in importance.

Today, the most common complaint of patients is that their doctors do not talk to them. A 1996 annual report of the complaints' committee of the College of Physicians and Surgeons of Ontario had to remind members that lack of effective communication had been at the crux of patient complaints since 1970. Patients need to talk about their illnesses and fears, often for a lot longer than their physicians or family members want to hear about them. In the literature on cancer patients, self-help groups and support groups have been identified as an effective and often the only coping strategy that helps people manage the emotional impacts of illness. And yet some doctors remain reluctant to refer patients to these non-medical sources of support. Patient frustration over the difficulties of finding support and information has now been eased by home computing and information technology, but this is no boon to the doctor-patient relationship when it brings the added burden of sorting through and making sense of piles of downloaded documents.

Patients are also assuming an increasing burden of the costs of care. In Canada, the privately-funded portion of health expenditures is second highest among G7 countries, and grew from 24% in 1975 to 31% in 1997. Taxpayers, patients and families are taking on a greater burden of cost and, because of this, can be expected to exercise consumer rights and preferences similar to our American neighbours. Neither can we ignore what is often called the "boomer" factor. The values of previous generations, shaped by the Depression and World Wars, embraced authority, security and conformity. The public respected the medical system and followed doctors' orders. In contrast, the formative experiences of baby boomers have been organized around education, civil rights, feminism, the environmental movement and the information explosion. Boomers are less deferential to authority, seek more information, involvement, choice and control. The consumer movement has also led to a dramatic increase in the development of self-help and advocacy groups. At the global level, an international alliance of patient organizations has recently emerged whose mission is to build health services with patients at their centre in every country. Parallel efforts are underway in Canada to establish a national patient advocacy coalition, and a summit has been convened for 1999 to build consensus toward the goal of establishing a patient-centred, patient-driven advocacy network.

Regaining public trust and confidence will require governments and the medical profession to reestablish a fundamental commitment to patients in the public's mind. Medical professionals and institutions have always sought to serve patients' needs, but have tended to rely on physicians to define those needs. This is no longer acceptable. We now need systematic efforts to incorporate patients' values and preferences into medicine, a change that could lead to a positive new role for the family doctor and to the realization that counseling is a crucial therapeutic tool. Time spent with patients is the essential element in making this change possible. If we want to revitalize and reinvent health care in this country and meet the actual needs of Canadians while doing so, we should be wary of implementing a technology-dominated system or, even worse, an efficiency-driven one. Instead, we need to put into effect a system that places greater monetary value on the time physicians spend with patients; a system that ultimately realizes the enormous therapeutic and social benefits resulting from such an approach.

Closing the Care Gap

Dr. Terrence Montague

The focus of health and disease management in Canada can be viewed as an evolution of paradigms, from the medicare paradigm originated in Saskatchewan 40 years ago to the cost-containment or restructuring paradigm implemented more recently across the country. In each paradigm, the drivers have been the same: access, cost and quality. When we first created medicare, the primary focus was on universal access, and that was appropriate. Decades later, we entered into a phase I experienced first-hand as Director of Cardiology at the University of Alberta: the era of restructuring, cost-containment and cost-efficiency, in which restriction of access was used as a major tool to achieve cost targets put in place by administrators. Now, we are at a crossroads, where many of us in the field hope to move towards an increased focus on quality and access in order to develop an evidence-based paradigm for managing health and disease. Quality and access in health care are of prime importance to all of medicare's constituencies. The Canadian public consistently indicate that the two are an overriding concern: physicians view both as key to improving health outcomes in major diseases across the population, and health administrators view their optimization as a way to lower costs without resorting to the restructuring we have seen previously.

However, changing a model is never easy, particularly in medicare, and if our health care paradigm is to now successfully shift from a cost-driven, restrictive paradigm to an evidence-based quality paradigm, much groundwork remains to be laid (Figure 1). In this light, my colleagues and I in the Patient Health Management Department of Merck Frosst Canada have developed a "recipe" for improving patient care and outcomes as we move to an evidence-based quality paradigm. For very burdensome diseases such as the cardiac diseases I am most familiar with, the recipe begins with the formation of a broad-based partnership between stakeholders includ-

Figure 1   *The Health Care Environment:*
A competing balance of driving forces

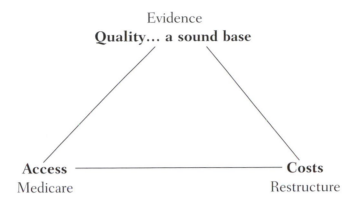

ing physicians, pharmacists, nurses, governments, and patients. The evidence base of optimum disease management involves more than just the knowledge about the efficacy of treatments we have gained from the great clinical trials of the last decade; there is now solid evidence that factors such as the comprehensiveness and seamlessness of care also drive quality outcomes, and that their absence decreases the quality of care. There is also evidence that the covenant between doctor and patient benefits outcomes, as shown in a large retrospective analysis done by the Clinical Quality Improvement Network (CQIN), which is a network of investigators interested in measuring care and outcomes among cardiac disease patients, which started in the West and now extends across Canada. When doctor and patient work together unimpeded to make treatment decisions, positive outcomes increase, even when there is no solid evidence that a particular treatment works. We must take all of these findings into account in any evidence-based approach.

CQIN also demonstrated the importance of measuring outcome variables and providing feedback to those involved in care. If you measure and provide feedback, the outcomes associated with what participants do will improve markedly. This is known as the Hawthorne Effect and it has tremendous applicability in health care, despite the fact that we do not know quite how it works. By measuring and providing feedback, you create a continuous quality improvement loop.

The Department of Patient Health Management at Merck Frosst Canada is putting this theory to work in a project called ICONS (Improving Cardiovascular Outcomes in Nova Scotia), begun approximately a year ago. The hypothesis is essentially that if we apply this recipe to cardiovascular diseases, we will see improved outcomes in the whole population at risk, and these outcomes will be as good or even better than those achieved in clinical trials. The design (Figure 2) involves repeated before and after measurements of specific interventions which will be designed by the steering committee. The make-up of that steering committee is one of the most important aspects of the recipe. This is health care renewal from the ground upwards, instead of from the top down.

Figure 2   *Creating a continuous quality improvement loop*

Process

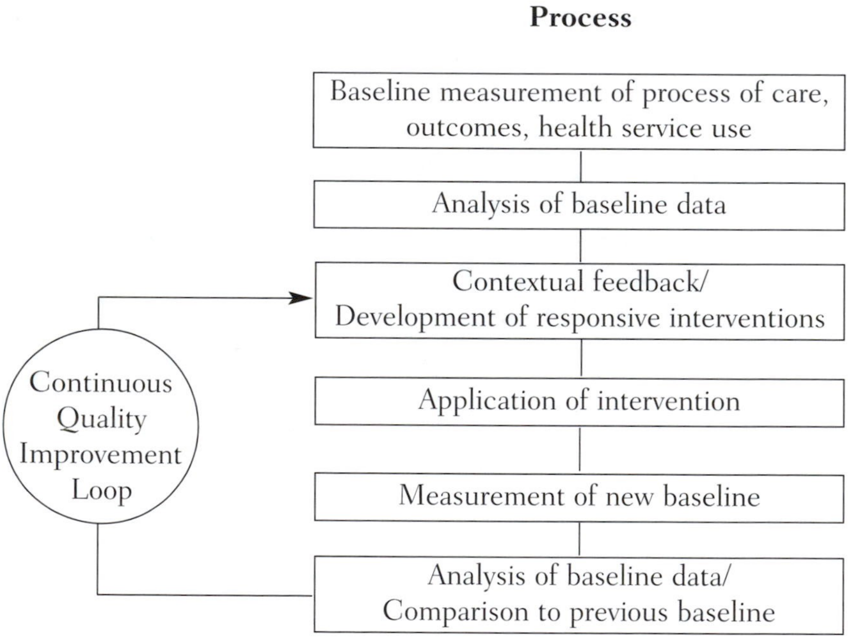

Source: *The Hospital Quarterly*, Fall 1998; Vol. 2, No. 1, p. 39.

ICONS' design is largely modeled on the National Institute of Health design governments use in large clinical trials. The steering committee are the principal investigators who drive the project and, in ICONS, they are drawn from each of the major communities in Nova Scotia. They include a general physician, a pharmacist, a community opinion leader, and a specialist, usually in internal medicine or cardiology. The outcomes that will be measured in this study are mortality, morbidity, costs, and utilization of proven and unproven therapies. The goal is to improve care, and the infrastructure put in place through this design stands a very high likelihood of markedly improving care and outcomes, particularly important outcomes like survival and hospitalization.

The ICONS design could be beneficial in other health areas as well, and Merck Frosst Canada's Patient Health Management Department is now forming partnerships in a variety of other initiatives. They all incorporate the same evidence-based principles, and focus on the gap that currently exists between best care and usual care. One such project is a proposed patient health program for the Province of Ontario, which is presently undergoing feasibility assessment. It is unique in that it proposes to manage groups of diseases, in this case diseases that are particularly prevalent among and important to women. There is a greater difference between usual care and best care for women than for men.

Irrespective of one's viewpoint as a patient, professional, care provider, regulator or product developer, the goal of health care is the same: the best care and the best outcomes for the most people at the best cost. The gap between efficacy evidence demonstrated in clinical trials and effectiveness in the population requires closing the circle of scientific progress from basic discovery to greatest human benefit. To this end, I suggest that using evidence-based quality improvement as a guiding principal provides the best chance of creating a sound clinical basis for health policy in the future.

Integrating Heart Care

Dr. Hugh Scully

The Cardiac Care Network (CCN) of the Province of Ontario was formed some nine years ago as a system put together by professionals, the public, hospitals and government to address the very real needs of patients requiring cardiac services in the province. To that end, therefore, it is patient focused: the sole objective is to enhance access to, and quality of, care. Data has been gathered, measured, monitored, evaluated, looked at objectively by third parties, and then brought into the debate with decision makers about how the money is to be spent.

There was a perception in the late 1980s and early 1990s, and I say "perception", that there were patients dying on waiting lists. At the time there was considerable public concern about the issue that could not be addressed because there was no objective way to assess patient urgency; there was a perceived lack of resources, but no centralized data, and only variable access to waiting list information. As well, there was no formal assistance for physicians wishing to refer patients who required care. It was at that point that the CCN was set up with a mandate to provide liaison and coordination for all adult cardiac patients, and to provide the Ontario Ministry of Health with information about how to make the best use of resources (Ontario has a separate pediatric cardiac system, with some integration between the two systems). Centres throughout the province have been involved in the network, eight of which are surgical and cardiac intervention centres.

The CCN developed a standardized system of information, based on an urgency-rating scale defined by consensus, to provide a level playing field for all patients and practitioners. The three facets of the triangle are patients, the referring doctors, and the cardiac centres (those tertiary centres that are difficult to comprehend and to gain access to), and the goal was to try and improve the communication and feedback loop. Coordinators have now been assigned to each centre to facilitate doctor to doctor communication. As a cardiac surgeon doing a lot of complex cardiac surgery, I can tell you that this last is a very critical issue. I rarely know who a patient's family physician is, never mind their community care giver. The establishment of this communication has been immensely helpful in building the family physician and the care givers in the community into the loop.

All patients are registered, and information about waiting times and other relevant matters is provided to patients and their families by both physicians and coordinators. Designed as a waiting list management system so that people could gain access to care within a reasonable time at minimal risk, the data is reported on a regular basis. Monthly and annual reports are published and made available on the Internet, to hospitals, and to family physicians. We now have very good information on referral patterns and on the prevalence of different forms of cardiovascular disease on a county by county basis. There seem to be some high risk areas of the province for coronary disease, although we have not yet determined the reasons why. While information is not currently collected on a provincial basis, it is collected in great detail in each of the institutions, and waiting times are balanced against urgency. In order to keep the information credible, reports from hospital coordinators and hospitals are later audited by people from outside the hospital.

Data is evaluated by the Institute for Clinical and Evaluative Studies in Ontario, providing a strong incentive to ensure that the data is honestly and accurately gathered and reported. Users, surgeons, referring doctors, hospital administrators, and CCN members including the public now all want to see the network expanded to include other aspects of cardiac care, like primary and secondary prevention and rehabilitation, so that there is integration of the community into this highly specialized area.

The CCN has been very effective in managing care. Research and planning have been accompanied by funding and accountability mechanisms that make each participant in cardiac care accountable to many others for their use of the system. One important feature is the emphasis on revising a patient's urgency rating scale if their condition changes, so that people do not fall through the cracks and, to the degree that we can prevent it, do not die on the waiting list. Public information on the Internet is being increasingly used by referring hospitals, referring doctors and by the public.

In 1996-1997, the mortality rate for people waiting for surgery was 0.74%; about 82 people. Of these 82 people, 80 would likely not have died had they had prompt attention. That number has been cut in half for the past year, results that are as good or better than any other system in the world right now.

Under the new system, the process of developing and situating new cardiac care centres has been of great interest. Professionals from all areas of expertise are afforded the chance to enter into discussion. This type of approach produces quick results: more patients waiting, more money infused, and the number of patients waiting comes down. There is enormous potential in informed debate. This exercise does not in any way conflict with a physician's responsibility to the individual patient as a surgeon, but instead takes advantage of his or her expertise to inform the debate, so that a rational decision is made. The government of Ontario has invested $65 million on the basis of recommendations received from the panel.

We have learned that the time between the heart study and surgery is the waiting period that really affects patients, not the time between seeing a specialist and surgery. Within all Ontario hospitals, urgent and semi-urgent cases are consistently treated within the time frame of three or four days recommended. The problem we have had is completing surgery within the recommended time for elective or non-urgent patients. While the median wait time has come down, it has not come down to a degree we are comfortable with, and certainly needs to be addressed further.

Reliable data lead to sound decisions, as does participation in a non-proprietary way by the leaders at the table, who include physicians, hospitals, government, and advocates for the public. We are working towards a national database, which is a partnership between Health Canada, the Heart and Stroke Foundation of Canada, and the Canadian Cardiovascular Society. The development of the Canadian Cardiovascular Database would represent the first time in the world that cardiac care givers together with government and the voluntary health sector have sat down and planned a system together.

Additional Thoughts on How Health Policy Can Respond to Clinical Imperatives

WHERE SHOULD RESOURCES GO?

Hugh Scully: It is very hard to put resources into public health when the public is demanding acute care in the emergency room because that is where their point of contact is. If there was more of a margin to maneuver in the system then we would be able to accomplish more.

Margaret Somerville: But it seems that the relationship with high tech is really what is driving expenditures at this time.

Richard Cruess: Dr. Scully is a high-tech doctor. I was an orthopedic surgeon, a high-tech doctor. The biggest waits are for total hip replacement and cardiac surgery. This is where public pressure is being applied.

Terrence Montague: One of the realities we face as health care providers in this country is that we live next door to the United States, the most medically high-tech society in the world, and that generates enormous expectations.

CHANGING PHYSICIAN ATTITUDES

Greg Robinson: Dr. Cruess talks about the window of opportunity that exists for the medical profession to make positive changes along the lines of the recommendations he suggests, chiefly through education. However, there is still a major difficulty, and that is the attitudes and behaviours that Dr. Cruess' recommendations do not or will not address.

Richard Cruess: I do not see any other way to address these issues other than through education in its broadest sense. Consequently, the first article that my wife and I wrote was addressed to the educational community.

Hugh Scully: In the list of competencies now articulated by the Royal College of Physicians and Surgeons in Canada and the College of Family Physicians in Canada, education in the areas that Dr. Cruess referred to are immediately addressed as part of the requirements for all training programs for physicians. Another hopeful development is the success of projects like the Cardiac Care Network. Doctors can work with others to realize positive change; it is just a matter of education within the profession as to how we can act as professionals and experts and make a positive difference where people count. That requires an educational process within the profession.

WHERE'S THE WIN?

Greg Robinson: How does Merck Frosst benefit from a project like ICONS?

Terrence Montague: Heart failure is a large public health burden. One percent of the country's total population suffers its effects and it has a very high morbidity and mortality rate. We have proven that medical therapy can improve the duration of life, but as a cardiologist, I began to realize that at best we were giving these proven therapies to only 50% of the people who could benefit from them, as opposed to 90% or even 100%. That discrepancy is what I call "the care gap." If we narrow or manage to close the care gap, the patient gets the benefit of the proven therapies, and pharmaceutical companies, like Merck Frosst, benefit from ensuring appropriate use of medications. In projects like ICONS, the design is accomplished by a steering committee, and there is no mandate to use particular products. Ultimately, closing the care gap benefits patients first and foremost, governments benefit by improving population health, and the companies which research and develop new technologies bene-

fit because the medications they produce reach the patients who
need them.

WHO DECIDES WHAT TREATMENT CAN BE OFFERED?

Robert Usher: I am concerned about the manner in which a doctor
is to make decisions about very costly care. In my field, which is
the care of premature babies, we could have to decide when it is
purportedly too costly to save the life of a 22-week gestation
baby with an uncertain outcome. Transplantation surgery is
another issue. Who should make these decisions?

Richard Cruess: The primary responsibility of the physician is to the
patient, and to keep himself or herself informed as to what the
most effective therapy is. It is, I think, wrong for a physician to
fail to inform a patient about the availability of a given form of
therapy simply because it is too expensive, all the while understanding that if that money comes out of the public purse, it will
mean less care for others in the system.

Some of those decisions have been made remarkably well,
and have involved the professional staff in medicine, nursing,
patients organizations and the board of governors of the institutions. When you are the individual's physician, I think it is your
responsibility to do your best to obtain therapy for that patient,
even if the system does not sanction it.

Hugh Scully: We feel the kind of tension Dr. Usher describes every
week in triage discussions. Do you decide to try new surgery on
a patient at very high risk, even if doing so will tie up the intensive care unit so that four or five other people won't be able to be
treated right away? I think the debate has to be taken beyond the
individual physician or group of physicians, so that society can
begin to participate in establishing priorities.

CHAPTER 3

Economic Considerations in Health Care

The Use and Misuse of Economics

Dr. Raisa Deber

Many discussions about health care justify universal, comprehensive coverage on grounds of "equity" and "Canadian values," but assume that hard-nosed economic considerations would instead justify a more U.S.-style "two-tier" model. Similarly, policy makers often tend to assume that Canadian spending for health care is somehow out of control, at least as measured against other industrialized countries. Closer examination reveals that both of these statements are myths, based on a misinterpretation of both the available data, and of economic theory.

Economics is called upon in discussions at all levels of health care, from the macro level of examining overall systems, to micro allocation issues of determining which services will be delivered to which individuals. This discussion concentrates on macro questions, beginning with an examination of international comparisons.

THE ECONOMICS OF INTERNATIONAL COMPARISON

Recent discussions about Canadian health expenditures have taken as their starting point the assumption that Canada is among the most expensive health care systems in the world. Canadian pride in medicare was easy to maintain when the basis of comparison was only the United States, which managed to spend more than any other country while still denying insurance coverage to a population greater than that of Canada. Once comparisons included other industrialized countries, however, analysts discovered that Canada appeared to be spending the second largest proportion of GDP for medical care, which would have given it the distinction of being the most expensive publicly-funded system in the world. The reaction was widespread shock, horror, and a determination to manage "out of control" spending; indeed, this "fact" is still widely cited to prove that Canada is spending "enough" for health care if only it could be better managed.

Recently retired health economist Jean-Pierre Poullier and his staff at the Organisation for Economic Cooperation and Development (OECD) have done a masterful job in attempting to standardize international data to allow these sorts of cross-national comparisons. Table 1 presents the health expenditures as a percentage of GDP for 22 OECD countries, in decreasing order, for 1993.[1] It was this table which helped to justify the cost-cutting furor we are now living through.

Table 1   *Health Expenditures 1993*

Country	% of GDP	Rank
U.S.	14.1	1
Canada	10.2	2
Germany	10	3
France	9.8	4
Switzerland	9.4	5
Netherlands	9	6
Sweden	8.9	7
Italy	8.6	8
Australia	8.5	9
Denmark	8.4	10
Finland	8.4	10
Iceland	8.3	12
Belgium	8.1	13
Norway	8.1	13
Austria	8	15
Portugal	7.7	16
Spain	7.5	17
Ireland	7.3	18
New Zealand	7.3	18
U.K.	6.9	20
Luxembourg	6.7	21
Japan	6.6	22

Source: OECD Health Data, A Comparative Analysis of 29 Countries, 1998.

As the table demonstrates, the United States spending, at 14.1% of GDP, was by far the highest, making everybody else look good. However, Canada ranked second, with 10.2%. In contrast, the U.K. spent only 6.9%. Japan appeared to be the model, spending only 6.6% of GDP for health care, while achieving excellent health outcomes. Panic ensued. What was Canada doing wrong? What was Japan doing right? And how should Canada reform its health care system to improve matters?

What few bothered to notice is that ratios do not just have numerators; they also have denominators. This point was first made by Robert G. Evans of the University of British Columbia in an article in Policy Options.[2] He began with the familiar chart comparing health spending as a proportion of GDP in the U.S., Canada, the U.K., and the average of all OECD countries. This data reveals that throughout the 1960s, Canada and the U.S. were spending virtually the same proportion of their economy for health care. From the early 1970s, these two lines began to diverge, with U.S. spending continuing to increase, and Canadian spending levelling out. Interestingly, 1971 marked the year in which all Canadian provinces had in place universal coverage for hospital and physician services, while the U.S. continued with its system of mixed financing, and this data was frequently used to argue for the superiority of universal coverage with a single payer. However, in the early 1980s, Canadian spending took a major jump. Evans noted that these years were associated with recession, and computed a hypothetical GDP series which would have applied had the Canadian economy continued to grow at the same rate it had between 1960 and 1980. The new chart depicting Canadian health expenditures as a proportion of this hypothetical GDP showed that it would have remained stable; indeed, the publicly-funded proportion (physician services and hospital care) would have decreased. Evans' analysis suggested that the key reason for the increase in Canadian expenditures as a proportion of GDP was problems in the denominator — that is, slow economic growth — rather than any inherent inefficiencies in the health care system itself.

Table 2   *Health Expenditures 1994*

Country	% of GDP	Rank	US $ per capita	Rank
U.S.	13.6	1	3628	1
Germany	10	2	2533	4
France	9.7	3	2230	7
Canada	9.6	4	1824	14
Switzerland	9.5	5	3508	2
Netherlands	8.8	6	1925	11
Sweden	8.7	7	1966	9
Australia	8.7	7	1592	15
Italy	8.4	9	1485	17
Iceland	8.1	10	1898	12
Belgium	8	11	1845	13
Austria	7.9	12	1943	10
Denmark	7.9	12	2297	6
Finland	7.9	12	1520	16
Norway	7.8	15	2222	8
Portugal	7.8	15	669	22
Spain	7.4	17	919	21
New Zealand	7.4	17	1056	20
Ireland	7.2	19	1073	19
Japan	7	20	2614	3
U.K.	6.9	21	1213	18
Luxembourg	6.5	22	2339	5

Source: OECD Health Data, A Comparative Analysis of 29 Countries, 1998

Table 2 illustrates the different ranks which arise from using different ways of measuring 1994 health expenditures. The data is taken
from the OECD database, the most recent year for which relatively
stable data exist. (Although the most recent OECD database includes
more recent data, this is provisional, and subject to revision.) The
countries are arranged in decreasing rank of spending as a proportion
of GDP. Again, the U.S. ranks first, although the most recent revision

puts their spending at 13.6% of GDP. Canada has dropped slightly, to 4th place, and Japan risen slightly, to 7% of GDP. But spending can also be measured in dollars per capita. The next columns show the rank and value of each country's actual spending in U.S. dollars per capita. The U.S. remains in first place. However, Canada's actual spending was $1,824 per capita, for 14th place. Japan, in contrast, was spending $2,614, in third place. Japan and Canada were thus mirror images in 1994 — Japan's relatively high level of expenditure nonetheless was a low percentage of its healthy economy, whereas Canada's moderate level of expenditures appeared high when its economy lagged, as it did throughout the 1980s. More details on different ways of measuring health expenditures can be found in papers prepared for the National Forum on Health by Arweiler[3] and Swan and Deber.[4,5]

The panic we have been living through as the "efficiency" of Canadian health care came under scrutiny thus appears to have been based in part on economic calculations that have been taken somewhat out of context. Spending as a proportion of GDP is obviously a crucial number, in that it reflects the carrying capacity of the economy and the opportunity costs of devoting these resources to health care. However, actual spending may be a better measure of whether things are "out of control." In the final analysis, none of these aggregate measures deal with the crucial questions of what services are being purchased, and with what effect. The efficiency of health care delivery — and there is always room for improvement in any system — is thus more a function of needs, incentives and organizational structures, than of these sorts of aggregate statistics, which provide little in the way of useful direction for health reformers. In particular, the international evidence provides little support for the commonly voiced assumptions that we "cannot afford" medicare. A more dangerous illusion, also sparked by that "second most expensive health system" myth is that public financing is inherently inefficient, and that following economic principles will lead us to allow a greater role for privately-financed care. All too often, supporters of ideas such as bringing in user fees for medically necessary services are justified in terms of a misapplication of the purported laws of economics.

Economic justifications for private health care

Consider the following two scenarios:

1) Someone comes into a hospital emergency room with a ruptured appendix, and no money. Should he be treated anyhow?

2) Suppose you were offered a free all-expenses-paid week for two in Hawaii (or Paris), with the only catch being that the trip had to be taken sometime within the next twelve months. Would you accept? Now, suppose you were offered free open heart surgery in an excellent teaching hospital, which must be taken within the next year? Would you accept?

And how do your answers to these questions accord with the laws of economics?

Economics deals with the distribution of commodities; Nobel Laureate Paul Samuelson has defined economics as "the study of how individuals and society choose, with or without the use of money, to employ scarce productive resources, which could have alternative uses, to produce various commodities over time and distribute them for consumption, now and in the future, among various people and groups in society."[6] In other words, economics deals with mechanisms for efficiently allocating scarce resources. Obviously, efficiency is not the only factor of importance in making resource allocation decisions; there are many things economics does not even try to address, including fairness, caring, and most of the other crucial aspects of life. But even if we take economics on its own terms, it soon becomes apparent that the basic principles underlying microeconomics do not apply very well when we are talking about medically necessary care.

In its simplest form, microeconomics deals with three components: supply, demand, and price. Price acts as the signaling factor that links supply and demand. Any self-respecting economist can plot supply and demand curves and look for their intersection. For example, if the price drops, demand should increase; there should be a near infinite demand for free goods. Conversely, if supply is fixed and demand is high, price should rise until enough people get priced out of the market to balance supply and this new (lower) level of demand at the new equilibrium price.

NEED AND USER FEES

However, these predictions do not accord well with the responses most people give to the two scenarios above. Consider Scenario 1: most people would treat the person with the ruptured appendix. In economic terms, this means that they would not allow him to be priced out of the market. Under those circumstances, we set up a rather peculiar economic model, in which there is a floor price (whatever charity or the public system will pay) but no ceiling price. The private tier is thus free to jack up their prices as high as they wish; anyone priced out of their market will simply fall back into the publicly-funded tier. Two disquieting consequences follow. First, as we have noted, market forces cannot act to achieve cost control. Second, however, the public tier will have to be inadequate (or at least, perceived as inadequate), or there would be no reason to pay extra for private health services. Contrary to the usual rhetoric about privately-funded care strengthening the public system by "freeing up" time and resources, a viable private tier depends upon eroding the publicly funded system. Not surprisingly, most studies have found a combination of higher costs and worse access (e.g., longer waiting lists) whenever mixed funding models are introduced; for a review of this material, see Deber et al's background paper for the National Forum on Health.[7]

Deber and Ross have suggested that one way of defining "medically necessary" care is in terms of our willingness to allow people to be priced out of the market. Assuming that a particular treatment is likely to be effective, is appropriate for the given condition, and is wanted by the potential recipient, society must determine whether it is willing to deny such care to those who could not afford to pay for it.[8]

In effect, there are three alternatives for people who "need" a service which they cannot afford to pay for themselves. The first is to buy the service anyhow; under this situation, people can and do spend themselves into bankruptcy, and are forced to make difficult choices (e.g., between food and medication). Under these circumstances, there is no cost control. Indeed, most health economists recognize that the reason why U.S. health care spending is so high is not because there are too few market forces operating, but because there are too many — cost control is achieved by denying care, rather than by otherwise constraining costs.

The second possibility is that people will decide to forego the service, either because they do not recognize it as necessary, or because they consider other things (e.g., food) to be of even higher priority. There is incontrovertible evidence that imposing a user fee will deter some utilization. Unfortunately, there is equally good evidence that this reduced utilization does not distinguish well between necessary and unnecessary visits. This is not really surprising, since if people had enough medical knowledge to distinguish between necessary and unnecessary visits, they would probably be doctors themselves. The deterrence effect is also far stronger for primary care than for the really expensive portions of the system (e.g., hospitalization), implying that savings are likely to be trivial. The deterrent effect of user fees is, not surprisingly, greatest for the people to whom the money matters the most — usually, the poor, the elderly, the sick, and the disabled. Indeed, utilization by those to whom the fee is trivial may increase, leaving total utilization (and costs) largely unchanged. To the extent that people seek care only when they are very sick, early detection, health education, and preventive medicine may go out the window. In addition to being lousy medicine, in many cases, this is also lousy economics. "Saving" money by restricting access to insulin for diabetics can generate costly hospitalizations and avoidable health problems.

The third possibility is that people would like to receive the care, and will seek assistance from others. An interesting ethical dilemma arises about whether society or charity will come to the rescue, or say "tough luck." If they come to the rescue, we move back to the first possibility and eliminate cost controls. If they do not, we move to the second possibility, and tell people that they are on their own.

A number of variations on user fees are often considered. For example, one proposal was to charge $5 per "unnecessary" emergency room visit, up to a maximum per patient, but with the fees waived for the poor or chronically ill. There are few administrators who would be able to administer this sort of scheme for less than the collection cost. In general, one suspects that all of the revenue collected by a "small" user fee would be required just to set up the administrative mechanisms required to collect it.

NEED AND UNNECESSARY CARE

But need has a flip side, as can be seen in considering the responses to Scenario 2. Most people would be eager to take that free trip to Hawaii. However, the offer of free surgery evokes laughter, followed by the condition, "only if I needed it." Microeconomics speaks of "demand." However, much of health care instead speaks the language of "need."

There is a category of good, often referred to as "merit goods," which most societies believe should not operate according to the laws of the market. Instead, these goods are allocated on some basis of need and merit. Need is a complex concept, and notoriously difficult to define. However, we tend to know it when we see it, at least in extreme situations. Market models are not designed to assist us in allocating resources on the basis of need. Indeed, the concept is inherently paternalistic, since "need" must be validated by some outside authority. I can tell you what I want, but we allow health professionals to determine what I need. And, just as we are unwilling to deny the man with the ruptured appendix care he "needed," we consider it inappropriate, or even unethical, to provide most medical services if they are not needed. If a shoe store has an excess supply, they may hold a sale, and no one worries if the buyer already has twelve pairs of similar shoes. However, if the Toronto Hospital had surplus operating room time, it could not advertise HALF-PRICE SURGERY, TODAY ONLY. We can speak of unnecessary surgery in a way we cannot speak about unnecessary shoes.

Clearly, not all goods offered as part of "health care" can be considered merit goods. Most people would be perfectly comfortable allowing people to be priced out of the market for cosmetic surgery. Indeed, certain services, particularly those in the "wellness" industry, can be purchased without reference to "need". We have little ethical problems if already fit people work out in a gym, and do not talk about "unnecessary" aromatherapy. Conversely, we probably feel that people with cancer should have access to appropriate chemotherapy. The mapping between what is currently covered under provincial health plans and what would be deemed "medically necessary" is thus good, but imperfect. Some rethinking is probably necessary if we are to continue to meet the basic compact between Canadians and their government — to ensure that high quality medically necessary care is accessible in a timely manner to all those who need it. In particular, there are certain services which probably should be publicly financed, and others which can be allocated using market approaches without doing violence to Canadian values, or to economic principles.

An impediment to this rethinking arises from the Canadian constitution. In 1867, when the country was formed, everything considered to be expensive and of national interest was made a federal responsibility, while everything considered to be cheap and of purely local interest was made the responsibility of the provinces. One of the responsibilities viewed as of purely local interest and assigned to the provincial governments was hospitals (grouped in with asylums, and charities). From that mention of the word "hospitals," the courts later decided that health care was a provincial responsibility, and now we are stuck with that decision. If we were designing a health care system from scratch today, we probably wouldn't make it a provincial responsibility; we would arrange some services at the local level, and others at regional or national levels. Certainly, a *de novo* system would recognize that Prince Edward Island or Manitoba would not have the population mass needed to support specialized services, such as pediatric cardiac surgery. Given the constitutional rigidities, and the differences in fiscal capacity across the country, universal coverage required that the national government take a role. Medicare grew up from "fiscal federalism"; the federal government agreed to provide some money to the provinces if they would comply with national terms and conditions. Medicare began with coverage for hospital care (in the 1957 Hospital Insurance and Diagnostic Services Act), and then added physician services (in the 1966 Medical Care Act). These terms and conditions were reaffirmed in the 1984 Canada Health Act. The national terms require the provinces to provide universal coverage for all medically necessary physician and hospital services, without co-payments to insured persons for insured services. But this restriction to the services covered under the previous legislation is becoming increasingly outdated. As technology allows us to provide care in the community, the rhetoric of reformers bumps up against the uncomfortable fact that moving care away from physicians and hospitals also moves it outside of the jurisdiction of the Canada Health Act. Any services outside the Act can be deinsured.

For this reason, the pharmacare and home care programs now being called for do not represent frills. Canada is increasingly using the move to the community to privatize the financing of care. As noted above, this trend makes little sense on either equity or economic grounds, as long as we are speaking about merit goods. It is essential to clarify and redefine what counts as care which we believe people should receive if needed, and to ensure that such care is publicly financed. Just as some surgery would qualify as a merit good, while other procedures might not, home care and pharmacare are not all-or-nothing propositions. There is no particular reason why we could not identify elements of home care and pharmacare that very much meet the criteria of merit goods and integrate those into the publicly funded health care system, while leaving public subsidy for other services, such as homemaking, to be carefully targeted (e.g., assistance in cleaning or meal preparation might be provided to low income individuals with functional limitations who are lacking social supports). These sorts of distinctions are unlikely to be simple; lines are rarely clear and cases rarely black and white. However, distinguishing between merit goods — which do not accord with the assumptions of market models — and other important goods which can nonetheless be allocated at least in part on the basis of market principles would not, I believe, undermine the moral basis of medicare.

The fact that standard economic concepts are not applicable to medically necessary services clearly implies the desirability of single-source, universal financing for such services. User fees or multi-tiered systems of financing for these sorts of services do not work, even in economic terms. Why, then, do people keep suggesting these approaches as a way of "saving" medicare? Bob Evans refers to such ideas as "zombies": ideas that should be dead, but keep getting up and going around doing damage.[9]

There are at least three reasons why we keep turning to zombies. One is ideological — believers in "free markets" find it difficult to rec-ognize situations when the underlying assumptions do not hold. One is political, springing from the recognition that costs are not borne equally. The first law of cost containment is: The Easiest Way to Cut Costs is to Shift Them to Someone Else. Governments are according-ly in a conflict of interest situation. As guardians of the public inter-est, they should ensure that necessary goods are financed in the most economically efficient manner, which would often imply public financing. But as payers, they also have strong incentives to shift costs out of their budgets, even if overall costs to the economy would rise. Indeed, to the extent that these additional costs would be borne by employers (through payroll expenditures for fringe benefits), a stronger reliance on private financing would also decrease economic competitiveness. However, these higher costs would not flow through government budgets. Similarly, providers would benefit from the abil-ity to evade cost controls, particularly if they could be assured that the public tier remained to guarantee that no one would be denied care. And the final reason is administrative — defining what would be defined as medically necessary is not an easy thing to do.

In background papers for the National Forum on Health, Eleanor Ross and I suggested something we called the "four-screen model" for deciding whether an intervention could be classified as medically necessary".[10] These screens would be applied sequentially. The first two screens are evidence-based. Screen 1 assesses effective-ness — does it work? Screen 2 assesses the likely benefit to the individual patient — is it needed? But screens 3 and 4 are based on values. Screen 3 assesses whether the intervention is wanted by the individual who might receive it. We suggested that if an intervention did not pass the first three screens, no one should pay for it. Screen 4 accordingly examines whether, given that an intervention was effective, appropriate, and wanted, the public should pay for it. A number of criteria might be used to decide, including economic effectiveness (cost minimization) and the need to foster research to clarify answers to earlier screens (e.g., to help determine effectiveness and appropriateness). A major determinant, however, would be this issue of merit goods — whether society would be willing to deny the intervention to those unable to pay for it. If the answer is "no", then no one could be priced out of that market, and public financing (along with other ways of controlling costs) would seem appropriate.

Although the four-screen model sounds very neat and manageable, it gets much messier when you try to put it into practice. The appropriateness and effectiveness of a type of care (the first two screens) can only be viewed on a sliding scale. Few things either work or don't; we must instead consider the likelihood of it working, the magnitude of benefit it brings. Deciding on the cut-off points where the effectiveness or appropriateness is "enough" will obviously be a matter of opinions and values.

Economic analysis is increasingly relied upon in making this type of micro allocation decision. Economic analysis often tries to finesse questions of values and priorities by attempting to disguise them as technocratic choices. These approaches also assume that human beings are always self-interested and always act rationally, both assumptions we intuitively know to be false. A cost-utility analysis might accordingly look at costs and consequences of a given treatment as compared to some alternative, and ask what it costs to buy an additional quality year of life, ignoring the conceptual problems in the way we currently measure health costs.[11, 12] The most widely accepted approach to establishing the economic benefit of some aspect of care — something called the "standard gamble" — confounds how we feel about risk with how we feel about outcomes. A standard gamble analysis will compute the value attached to a particular health state by asking how much additional risk of death one would be willing to run to avoid that health state. The point at which one is indifferent between the gamble and the health state is taken as the "utility" of that health state. For example, if one would be willing to try a surgical intervention with a 10% risk of death in order to avoid paralysis, but becomes indifferent when the surgical risk rises to 30%, the value of a year living paralyzed is deemed to be worth 0.7% of a normal life year. Now consider the example of a woman with cancer who is willing to put up with some rather horrific side effects to gain the possible survival benefits from aggressive chemotherapy. If she answers the standard gamble by indicating that she would not be willing to take any increased risk of death to avoid the side effects (that is, she wants maximum survival benefit), the analysis concludes that the quality of life on chemotherapy has the same value to her as living in perfect health, and that there would be no "quality improvement" from finding a milder form of therapy. This downplays all concern for comfort and quality. The approach also runs into some questions around how we treat time, how we view long-term and short-term effects and outcomes, and how we consider an individual decision as opposed to a collective decision. Economic approaches are vulnerable to charges of discrimination and they can be seen as immoral; as well, they focus only on the ends and not on the means used to accomplish these ends. However, economic analyses are simple to compute and provide deceptively precise estimates which are much appreciated by people who are trying to make decisions. They also have the merit of being explicit about the assumptions being made.

One classic example of the purported failure of these sorts of economic evaluations occurred in Oregon, which attempted to define which interventions would be insured for its Medicaid (poor) population, based on complex mathematical computations derived from this type of economic analysis. The results were counter-intuitive, and revised lists were eventually used. However, a study by Weinstein and Teng revealed that the computations had been done incorrectly; indeed, the values determined by the Oregon process did not correlate at all with other published cost-effectiveness analyses for the same procedures.[13] The failure points out this key advantage — the analysis was sufficiently explicit that researchers were able to identify precisely where they had gone wrong!

The philosopher of science, Abraham Kaplan, wrote about what he termed "the law of the instrument" — if a child is given a hammer, she will soon decide that everything is a nail.[14] By the same token, economics can give us extraordinarily useful tools to analyze the best way of allocating scarce resources to achieve a given goal. But, it can do so if, and only if, the underlying assumptions are sufficiently valid. Economics can't tell us what goals are important, particularly when dealing with things we consider medically necessary. Blind use of market approaches, like the blind use of managerialism so well critiqued earlier by John Ralston Saul, will often act much as Kaplan's hammer would in trying to repair a delicate and expensive watch. A more delicate touch would seem to be required.

End notes

1. Organisation for Economic Co-operation and Development. OECD Health Data. Compact Disc: "A Comparative Analysis of 29 Countries," 1998.

2. Evans R.G. "Health care reform: the issue from hell." *Policy Options 1993*: 14(6):35-41.

3. Arweiler, D. "International comparisons of health expenditures." In: National Forum on Health, ed. *Striking a Balance: Health Care Systems in Canada and Elsewhere*. v.4. Sainte-Foy, Quebec: Éditions MultiMondes, 1997.

4. Deber, R.B., Swan, B. "Puzzling issues in health care financing." In: National Forum on Health, ed. *Striking a Balance: Health Care Systems in Canada and Elsewhere*. v. 4. Sainte-Foy, Quebec: Éditions MultiMondes, 1998:307-42.

5. Deber, R.B., Swan, B. "Canadian health expenditures: myths and realities in the 'cost crisis'." CMAJ in press.

6. Samuelson, P.A. *Economics. An Introductory Analysis*. 7th ed. New York: McGraw-Hill Book Company, 1967.

7. Deber, R.B., Narine, L., Baranek, P., et al. "The public-private mix in health care." In: National Forum on Health, ed. *Striking a Balance:*

Health Care Systems in Canada and Elsewhere. v. 4. Sainte-Foy, Quebec: Éditions MultiMondes, 1998: 423-545.

8. Deber, R.B., Narine, L., et al. Op. cit.
9. Evans, R.G. "U.S. influences on Canada: can we prevent the spread of Kuru?" In: Deber, R.B., Thompson, G.G., eds. *Restructuring Canada's Health Services System: How Do We Get There From Here?* Toronto: University of Toronto Press, 1992:143-8.
10. Deber, R.B., Narine, L., et al. Op. cit.
11. Gold, M.R., Siegel, J.E., Russell, L.B., Weinstein, M.C., eds. *Cost-Effectiveness in Health and Medicine.* New York: Oxford University Press, 1996.
12. Deber, R.B., Goel, V. "Using explicit decision rules to manage issues of justice, risk, and ethics in decision analysis: when is it not rational to maximize expected utility? *Med Decis Making* 1990; 10(3): 181-94.
13. Tengs, T.O., Meyer, G., Siegel, J.E., Pliskin, J.S., Graham, J.D., Weinstein, M.C. "Oregon's medicaid ranking and cost-effectiveness." *Med Decis Making* 1996; 16(2): 99-107.
14. Kaplan, A. *The Conduct of Inquiry: Methodology for Behavioral Science.* Scranton, PA: Chandler Publishing Company, 1964.

Where Does Economics Belong in Health Policy: Three Views

Who Bears the Burden of Quebec's Universal Drug Plan?

Nathalie St-Pierre

Mixing economics and public health policy can form a dangerous cocktail. Quebec's new universal drug insurance plan, brought in two years ago, highlights the difficulties of reconciling economic imperatives with health policy. I will examine Quebec's drug plan in this light, and look at where the economic burden of the plan now falls.

The idea of a drug insurance plan was first suggested by the Hall Commission in 1964, and was proposed again by the Castonguay-Neveu Commission in 1970. After 30 years of pressure from various public interest groups, the government finally agreed to consider a plan in 1996, although by then there was good reason to suspect that the welfare of health consumers was not the government's chief concern. The decision was made during a period of high public debt and increasing poverty across Canada and in Quebec especially. Medical expenses were spiralling just as transfer payments were falling, and "rationalization" was the order of the day.

In the first half of the 1990s, Quebec's health services sector had seen some 13,300 jobs vanish, with seven hospitals closing in Montreal alone. By 1995, the cost of drugs as a proportion of health spending had increased to 11.8%, the highest in Canada at the time. The principal objectives of the Quebec government in introducing a public insurance scheme were threefold: to cover the 1.2 million Quebeckers then uninsured; to safeguard jobs in the private insurance sector; and to do it all without costing the government extra money. Research was commissioned to estimate the costs of various approaches.

The 1996 Castonguay report offered three options (Table 1), all of which increased the burden dramatically for welfare recipients and senior citizens, but promised to cut between $250 million and $410

Table 1 *Individual contributions in the various universal drug insurance plan proposals*

OPTION →	Castonguay Report 1996				
	Option A	Option B	Option C	Bill 33	Law 1996
Premium	$176	$83	$118	$176	$175
Premium for children	$0	$100	$0	$0	$0
Premium for adults	$100	$1,000	$500	$100	$100
Copayment	20%	10%	10%	25%	25%
Ceiling	$1,000	$2,000	$1,000	$750	$750

million from the government's share of the bill. An internal study, the 1995 Gagnon report, was also reviewed by the government but never acted upon. The report proposed dramatically reducing drug expenses for most citizens, but would have cost the government an extra $600 million annually.

BILL 33: A MIDDLE OF THE NIGHT SOLUTION

The Quebec government largely ignored the expert reports it had commissioned, and instead developed legislation without serious prior consultation. The new law was passed as Bill 33 and was immediately imposed on seniors and welfare recipients, the two groups slated to face the largest hike in drug expenditures under its provisions. Six months later, in January 1997, the legislation was extended to cover the entire population of the province.

Whereas welfare recipients had previously received prescription drugs for free, the new plan saw this group now contribute an annual total of $90 million to the province's drug bill. Seniors, who had hitherto paid $42 million, saw their total contributions rise to $275 million. Citizens outside these special groups who had previously been uninsured saw their costs rise slightly from $193 million to $203 million, while those who already had insurance faced a similar small rise, from $783 million to $821 million. Meanwhile, the government's share of the burden toppled from $922 million to its current level of about $551 million.

The new plan called for premiums to be based on income, rising to an upper limit of $175 a year, and included a deductible applicable whenever drugs were purchased. The deductible was originally proposed as 20% of the cost of the drug, but was then raised to 25% to discourage the population from "shopping around" for prescribed drugs.

COST-SHIFTING ONTO THE POOR

A drug is not a regular commodity or luxury good that needs financial disincentives attached to its purchase. When a physician prescribes a necessary drug for a patient, health concerns leave the latter little choice as to purchasing the medication. As a result, it is vital that policy-makers consider the socioeconomic status of their populations when undertaking economic and health policy reforms like the drug plan. At the time the Quebec plan was implemented, there was clear evidence that it was the poor who needed drug insurance most. Seventy percent of those with above-average incomes have private insurance; the figure drops to about 15% among the poor. In passing on the costs to this vulnerable group, the government failed to address the key values of who should get what at what cost.

Under the plan, a person who earns under $12,000 a year could spend 6.7% of their income on prescription drugs. For someone earning more than $30,000 a year and taking the same medication, however, the expense represents only 1.5% of their income. A retired person who had no costs beyond $2 user fees before the plan, could now pay $275 annually, plus one-quarter the cost of each prescription.

The Quebec drug plan has now been in effect for two years, and it has become clear that the system is neither fair nor equitable. Simply stated, people in lower income brackets have to spend too much for what they get in return. In response, some are even cutting back on their costs by rationing the use of the drugs they need. This cannot be good for public health, and may even rebound on the cost-cutters in terms of more hospitalizations.

If there is a lesson to be drawn from Quebec's experience, it is that policy-makers must identify at the outset what it is that they are trying to accomplish, as well as which segment of the population they are trying to affect or protect. The public must then be invited and encouraged to participate in effectively debating proposals before they become policy. In the case of Quebec's universal drug insurance plan, the provincial government disregarded input from experts and the public alike, and then developed policy ensuring that the government itself was the intended beneficiary of its own legislation. At the end of the day, the province is the only party involved which has seen costs go down. In a more democratic process, this would surely have been unacceptable and Quebeckers would not have the flawed plan they do today.

Changing the Idea of Value in Economics

Dr. Devidas Menon

Raisa Deber suggested earlier in this chapter that economists are usually advocates of cost containment, and cost-containment in health care often ends up meaning cost-shifting. This in turn can lead to multiple tiers, user fees, and other undesirable developments. While I do not disagree with that analysis, it is perhaps not quite fair to blame all of this on the science of economics. Cost-containment is a strategy, and if government chooses to adopt that strategy, then economics can help by providing the analytical tools to better implement that policy. But those same tools can be equally useful in implementing other kinds of policies. As well, economists are now developing analytical methods which do incorporate variables like the patient's preferences and quality of life issues. Moreover, it is fair to ask just how much the decision-making processes we use today in health policy take equity into account.

A SET OF TOOLS

It is an inescapable fact in modern health care that we cannot do everything we would like to for everyone. We should view economics as a set of tools that can help us make tough choices, and perhaps we should concentrate on funding services that are medically necessary and demonstrably effective, and worry less about more peripheral services. This is less an attempt at cost-containment than a cost-effectiveness strategy, and cost-effectiveness is surely a good thing.

Remembering always that economics is not a value-free discipline, it is worthwhile to ask what it can contribute to health policy making. Most of the work being done today in health economics is in economic evaluation. Through economic evaluations health policy can be better developed to incorporate the concept of value for money. It may seem crass to refer to value for money in health care, but it must be remembered that value does not have to be monetary. We can define value any way we like. Health status and mortality rates are two obvious ways in which the value of a particular health policy might be measured.

DATA NEEDED

The people whose job it is to manage and spend public funds on health care have to use value-for-money comparative methods, or they are not measuring the impact of their policy. There has been a lot of talk about how medicare is underfunded, and how it will probably require a bigger slice of our GNP, or greater per capita expenditure.

But nobody is asking what value, what outcomes, the current level of spending is buying. We need more health data and more economic data to tell us about cost and utilization of health services and the outcomes they are achieving. We also need to ensure such data are reliable and accurate.

In some provinces, governments are trying to set up large computerized health information systems; Alberta's WellNet project is one such example. The hope is that the large amounts of data generated by these systems will eventually enable governments to make better informed policy decisions. Economic information can make choices and assumptions explicit, and can permit different options to be compared based on the value for money they might offer. That value for money can then be taken as one element in the final decision-making process.

In Canada today, the pharmaceutical industry plays a leading role in economic evaluation. Provincial governments sometimes require drug companies to provide economic evaluation data as a prerequisite to getting their drugs put on formulary. At the same time, the process of economic evaluation is becoming broader and more inclusive. How, for example, do you compare the benefits of a new health-care program to those of a new education program? Recently, economists have been tackling this kind of problem with some success. It is all very well to say we should pour more funding into a certain avenue of health research, but that money is coming from somewhere, and we should try to know beforehand who is going to bear that cost. What reduction in service will there be in one area if costs go up in another? These are the kind of questions that economic evaluation can answer.

FROM KNOWLEDGE TO ACTION

Having the information is a good first step, but we also need mechanisms to turn information into action. There is little point in performing economic evaluations if there is no receptive audience for them among policy-makers. Better communication must be established between those who provide information and those who must act on it. Health economics research is a process, not just a series of steps, and the final stage of that process should be concrete proposals for action.

While policy-makers could benefit from a greater understanding of health economics, economists must recognize that policy-makers sometimes reach sensible decisions that are not necessarily rational decisions. There will always be other, overriding principles involved.

Perhaps the best definition of the role health economics can play in health policy formulation comes from the most recent issue of the British journal *Health Economics*. In it, Alan Maynard, an economist from York in England, and Cam Donaldson of the University of Calgary, review the work in health economics of the last 25 years and conclude as follows: "Hopefully in the next 25 years, researchers will improve their methods, and work better with future colleagues, to explore the intriguing areas so far subjected to rigorous analysis in only a limited manner. After much methodological advancement in particular areas, and vigorous evangelism by some of its practitioners, economics is permeating the formation of health policy increasingly at macro and micro levels. It has much more to offer in providing an understanding of policy issues and individual and institutional behaviours."

"Hopefully, we are gradually moving to an era of evidence-based policy making, where decisions about issues such as 'rationing' and health care reform will be informed by a knowledge base rather than by rhetoric and ignorance." Health economics can help achieve this.

Economic Analysis in the Policy-Making Process: An Inside Look

Dr. John Wade

During a two-year period of psychosis, I was a Deputy Minister of Health in Manitoba, an experience that allows me to describe what life was like in a turbulent provincial health ministry and what it may be like in the near future. The ministry's mission was to preserve, protect, and if possible improve the health of Manitobans. It is always easy to admit that grandiose missions in government are part hallucination, but we should not minimize their impact and importance: keeping long-term goals and values in mind is vital when one is plowing through the day-to-day activities of governance. At the time of my appointment, Manitoba was in a process of transformation from the hospital and doctor-based health system enshrined by Tommy Douglas to a more balanced program that took into account other determinants of health. The program was rapidly growing to encompass long-term care, home care, pharmacare, and palliation, among other concerns, and the health ministry had to grapple with the escalation of these types of services.

Like all other governments in Canada at the time, we were also faced with a large deficit. The Manitoba government was dealing ruthlessly with this deficit, and consequently a lot of health policy was determined not in the health ministry but at the Manitoba treasury board. Similarly, while the government was advocating a transition from a resource-based to a knowledge-based economy, it was hammering educational facilities with cutbacks authorized by the treasury board deficit-reduction program. Faculties of medicine and health sciences were among the victims, despite the fact that, overall, they account for about 60% of the research going on in Canada's universities.

More recently, Canadians have learned that the provinces of Manitoba, Alberta and Saskatchewan have balanced their budgets, and that more money will be available for health care. Government's main concern is now to decide how this money will be spent, a process that necessarily involves setting up mechanisms to determine where and how new funds can best be used. During my time in Manitoba, we tried to make sure that policy formulation was always based on the best possible information. To this end, we created the Manitoba Centre for Health Policy as a joint venture between government and Manitoba's universities. The Centre has an independent board and the ability to publish independently in peer-reviewed journals. It is free to comment and make criticisms publicly, and can keep tabs on what the health ministry does or doesn't do. This arrangement ultimately benefits both government and the public in its ability to influence the appropriate dispersal of funds for health care.

Manitoba has compiled comprehensive medical records from physicians and hospitals over two decades. This knowledge base has been enriched in recent years with help from Revenue Canada to include socioeconomic data, pharmacare data, public health data, and information from the fields of education and justice. The province also formed a partnership with the Royal Bank of Canada to bring information to doctors' offices and emergency clinics where it could be easily accessed. The usage of medical data banks raised important issues of confidentiality, and new legislation was passed to address these concerns. Technical measures were also taken to preserve data security.

In Manitoba, the health ministry tried to build a picture of health status against which to judge the impact of new policies. To establish this baseline, the ministry went beyond basic accounting procedures and the simple counting of operations, and split the province into ten regions based on postal codes. Family services, public health, home care and similar resources were divided between the regions. Tertiary care was not included because the patient volume was too small for such a division to work effectively. Similarly, the population of Manitoba is too small for some services to be effectively subdivided at the provincial level, a situation that led the ministry to form a Western Canada consortium for pediatric cardiac surgery. A similar approach might be advisable in areas like transplants and diagnostic imaging.

MAKING CARE ACCESSIBLE
ACROSS THE RURAL-URBAN DIVIDE

We often hear that the distribution of doctors in Canada is driven by treasury boards and fiscal imperatives, and not by the population's needs. This is true to some extent. People complain that because of this factor there are too many doctors concentrated in cities, but if we look at the inner core of Winnipeg, we discover instead that there are not enough doctors in the areas with the poorest health status.

This is not to deny that rural Canada is understaffed. Canada has had a two-tier health care system for many years, with the rural sector losing out. Most provinces have not put the funding for family practitioners out into the regions. Tertiary care has to remain centralized, of course, but for primary care should be distributed in the regions, as at the end of the day, physicians will go where the money is.

In the far North, private sector physicians did not want to deliver care to remote areas, so the Faculty of Medicine at the University of Manitoba founded the Northern Medical Clinic, now called the Northern Health Unit. We trained nurse practitioners but brought in surgery, and most of perdiatric surgeries performed in Churchill are actually performed by the best surgeons in the province. The University chose this avenue, rather than training a general practitioner to be all things to all people, so that it could maintain an active presence in the community. This approach enabled us to become advocates for better water, sewage and housing, and permitted us to identify with the community to a greater extent. As a result, we have now seen about 20 local aboriginal people become doctors, nurses and dentists in their home area.

EFFICIENCY AS AN ATTAINABLE GOAL

Cases for and against an approach based on efficiency, particularly cost efficiency have been stated in previous sections of this book. While every area of concern is different, the statistics that we in Manitoba compiled on cataracts, for example, seem to suggest that efficiency is not just a chimera but a real and attainable goal. In cardiology, we have coped with a 70% increase in coronary bypass operations. None of the credit belonged to the Manitoba government: instead, it was the health care providers on the front lines who made the system better by doing more with the same resources. Elective coronary surgery is now done with same-day admission, and the vast majority are discharged within four days. Only 10% of patients go into intensive care afterwards.

In a time of significant cutbacks to the Manitoba health care system, the mortality rate following major surgical procedures stayed stable or even dropped. Morbidity rates also went down, when readmission was used as a marker, as did visits to emergency wards by patients who had undergone major surgery. If patients had been discharged too soon one would expect readmissions to go up; the fact that they did not seems to indicate that hospitals had previously been hanging on to patients' stays unnecessarily.

When 400 beds were cut from the Manitoba system, research showed that only 50% of persons admitted to hospitals actually needed to be there. The other half could easily have been treated as outpatients or by home care, as Manitoba has a very good, though limited, home care system. Research in Saskatchewan by Stephen Lewis and his colleagues has found the same pattern.

This is certainly not to suggest that health care systems such as Manitoba's have enough resources. Rather it is a testament to the Herculean efforts of health care providers and managers, who have stretched limited resources to achieve maximum effect, often at considerable personal cost to themselves. Governments are saving money, but the price is paid by doctors, managers and especially nurses — a state of affairs reflected in the current flight of Canadian nurses to the United States. Health care providers are still working far too hard under far too much stress.

TARGETING CARE

I would agree strongly with Nathalie St-Pierre that anyone responsible for health spending decisions must first consider the target population and its health status. These considerations necessarily extend to health promotion and disease prevention as well as acute care. If one looks at the wealthiest part of Winnipeg, one finds an average of about 400 hospital days per 100,000 resident per year. But in the poorest parts of the city, this figure is about three or four times higher, at over 1,000 hospital days per 100,000 residents per year. The obvious question is, would money be better spent on health promotion in these poorer areas than on acute care?

The difficulties experienced by the aboriginal community poses one such problem in Western Canada, but the sensitivity and complexity of the subject makes it essentially taboo in policy-making circles. Aboriginal peoples in Manitoba make up 12% of the province's population, but account for 25% of births, 50% of children in pediatric hospitals, and 75% of children in the care of family services. Most of the young men in Manitoba's jails are of aboriginal origin. The health status of the aboriginal community is clearly far worse than that of the general population, but nobody wants to talk about the problem, let alone spend money on it. Aboriginal patients are not represented by health advocacy groups or policy-makers and providers, yet their circumstances ensure they place the greatest demands on the health care system.

IMPROVING HEALTH CARE

Political considerations always play a big role in the management of health care. If funds are injected into the system in an election year, will they be spent on large-scale public health problems like those experienced by Manitoba's aboriginals, or used to open more hospital beds and emergency rooms? The first option may be of more benefit to the health of the population, but the latter is ultimately the better vote-winner. Nowadays health policy decision-makers are often faced with overt political pressure from the highest levels, as well as from spin doctors worrying about how it will all look in a ten-second television clip.

Unfortunately, our present system of government is not structured to deal with health issues or indeed any issues in a holistic manner. Instead, health care is divided into discrete silos, often competing against each other for funds rather than solving problems. Only politicians with new ideas can break the pattern. When we tried in Manitoba to involve family services and the education department in health policy, our ministry had a series of running battles with the treasury board over accountability, despite the fact that many difficult health problems can only be addressed with a multi-departmental approach. In the case of diabetes, which now affects about 40% of aboriginal women, any effective program needs input from the ministry of agriculture (to try and find alternatives to junk food), as well as advice about encouraging physical exercise, and other concerns outside the purview of a typical health department. Currently, our governmental system just is not set up to administer programs multilaterally.

Despite having delivered acute care all my life, I am very conscious of the fact that there are other ways to improve people's health status which are not being given enough attention. I am currently involved in developing policy for physician remuneration in Ontario, and I find that our means of measuring doctors' performance are often completely removed from a context involving patients. When I was a practitioner in the far North and in rural Alberta, most of my day was not spent doing evidence-based medicine. Instead, I found myself talking to my patients, advising them, and sometimes consoling them. These imponderables are never measured, yet they are a crucial part of patient-doctor interaction. As we design new remuneration systems, we need to take these factors into account, not just for physicians but for all health care providers. We are entering a new era, at least in western Canada, where we will again have money to spend on health care. Let us make sure we spend it wisely.

Additional Thoughts on the Assumptions Behind the Numbers

THE BURDEN OF ILLNESS

Rachel Miller: Several years ago I wrote a publication on the economic burden of illness in Canada, which basically took the national health expenditure and attempted to break it down by disease category. I found it very frightening that we are still largely unable to answer basic questions about what different health problems are costing us. Fortunately we are now starting to include this cost of illness data when planning for the allocation of limited resources. Obviously the "What is he paid?" approach is imperfect, but at the same time, putting some sort of value on life is better than giving it none at all and simply counting hospital costs and doctors' bills as the whole impact of a disease.

Raisa Deber: Burden of illness statistics are valuable so long as we do not forget how much these numbers depend on what we decide to include as a cost. My favourite example of dubious cost of illness estimates is one the tobacco industry put out in which they decided that once a person reaches 65 they become a cost to society because they are not producing, they are collecting pensions. The inference was that the tobacco industry are society's benefactors, because they are killing people off just as they become "unproductive," thus reducing the net cost of illness. There is also the question of lost productivity estimates, which go against some of our basic values in the way they assume that the death of a high earner is worse than the death of a low earner. There are some rather insidious assumptions that can creep in when we start to put numerical figures on the value of people's lives. In a country with 10% unemployment, most people can easily be replaced in the work force, so those kinds of estimates could easily conclude that their death is not really a loss to productivity.

John Wade: Burden of illness studies are valuable, however, in alerting people to a disease that is consuming a disproportionate amount of national resources. This is particularly the case if a preventive, rather than acute, treatment approach can save money. Burden of illness statistics can be used to persuade employers, for example, to invest in prevention out of enlightened self-interest.

Margaret Somerville: We must be careful with this line of thought, however, because we spend health care money not just to get what we buy in terms of the provision of health care itself, but also because of the values we want to preserve. Why do we spend millions on air-sea rescue for one person lost at sea when we often will not spend a few thousand to put up road barriers that could save dozens of lives? The reason is that these economic decisions reflect different levels of threat to the societal value of respect for human life. The former is much more of an assault to this than the latter. What we are really talking about in deciding on funding for the health care system is a combination of two things: what health care we will and not provide, and our respect as a society for the intrinsic value of each human life. As a society, we cannot afford to forget health care carries this value.

Public, private, or charitable?

Diane Lister: We have heard a great deal about the off-loading of costs by government, and about cost-containment, but nothing about the role of the not-for-profit sector as a partner both in planning and in funding. There are some interesting statistics that should perhaps be brought into the discussion. Last year in Canada, the charitable sector generated a total of $86 billion. Our foundation grants about $20 million annually to the Hospital for Sick Children, representing about 10% of its operating budget. A survey we conducted in the greater Toronto area for the academic health sciences teaching hospital looked at the endowment campaigns planned over the coming three years. We found there was an aggregate total of $1.2 billion being sought in that one region, mostly to fund medical research.

It is important that we decide what a tax-based system should fund and what philanthropists should fund. And since citizens are giving the money, how can we involve them in decisions on where it goes? This is a large sector that is just not being recognized.

Nathalie St-Pierre: Leaving everything to the personal choice of individuals would be a retrograde step. People need to have confidence in government's ability to make the right decisions on spending. If people lose that confidence, it explains the growing role of the charitable sector. I think we must make government accountable for what it does and for where the tax money goes.

John Wade: This is certainly an issue in provinces that are moving towards regionalization. There is a temptation to get rid of the previous hospital board, as we have recently seen done by the hospital authority in Alberta. When we created the Winnipeg Hospital Authority we chose to leave the boards in place and not to interfere with the hospitals' particular traditions and cultures. Most of all, we wanted to leave in place not just the fund-raisers, but the volunteers who give the institution its character, and contribute so much to their efficient operation. It is important to leave the board intact, and with them the citizen participation.

Raisa Deber: Charitable groups can do more than just ease the burden on the public system. Because they can set their own agendas, they can work in otherwise neglected areas, introducing, for example, new ideas in health promotion. If they are successful, government may step in later on and pick up the bill. There is also an enormous amount of labour that charities provide along with funds. There is a lot of work done charitably that I do not think the system could manage without. The equation "government OR not-for-profit" misses that critical part of the issue.

Jim Armstrong: One might ask whether there would be a sounder basis for health care's future if the private proportion of our expenditure was reduced. Of course that would demand further resources from the public sector, and higher taxes to get the kind of health care system we want.

Nathalie St-Pierre: Quebec's experience with the crisis in the private sector indicated that there should probably be less private involvement in health care. Obviously that means higher publicly-borne costs, which will have to be distributed fairly. If we keep in mind that Canadians value their health care system, I think they are capable of deciding what is needed and who should be covered. We would come up eventually with an equitable system that provides good care. The discussion has to be held on a more open basis and it should include the people who will be directly affected.

Raisa Deber: There is a difference between financing care and delivering it. In terms of delivery, we do not have a public health care system in Canada. What we call public hospitals are in fact private, they are simply not-for-profit. And when we talk about private, we should distinguish between not-for-profit and for-profit organizations. In terms of financing, the real question is less "public" vs. "private" than "What do I have to pay, and what do I get in return?" If public schools are so bad that I have to send my child to private school, or if public transport is so bad that I have to use toll roads, these are deductions from my income, even if they do not appear as taxes. The same is true if I have private health insurance that costs three times as much as I would pay for publicly-funded health care. These things cannot be assessed by just comparing levels of taxation.

I am not sure we need more total money in the health system, but we do need to pay some attention to how it is allocated. Right now we have a system replete with perverse incentives. Why, for instance, can we not have a registry like the Cardiac Care Network that Hugh Scully described, rather than leaving doctors to phone around desperately looking for a bed or a specialist? With a certain amount of, dare I say it, good management, we could surely make more of the resources go where they need to be.

CHAPTER 4

Political Considerations in Health Care

Health Policy in the Consumer Era

The Honourable Bob Rae

Politicians are always the villains of the piece. There is a populist rhetoric that creates two different species: human beings and politicians. It is easy to blame others for our problems, but the issues politicians face are public issues that all of society has to confront. Public opinion, however, is often contradictory. Public opinion surveys uninformed by the larger world outside health care won't tell you much about the nature of public choice and political options. Governing is inevitably about choice, and choice requires that we do some things and not others. We can't, for instance, talk of spending more money on health care without also talking about taxes or holding back on other areas of spending.

There is currently a lot of talk of pouring money back into health care. More money without a better plan is a waste of money. From my time in government, I believe that as profoundly as I believe anything. If you ask the public whether they are concerned about the future of health care and want governments to spend more money on it, the answer will invariably be "yes". If you ask people if they and their doctors should be the only ones involved in deciding on treatment, the answer will also be "yes". But at some point you have to realize that none of these are very hard questions. Everyone wants to have their cake and eat it, and they want the same amount of cake to be left after they finish. This is just a fact of life. Canadians want European-style services and American-style taxes, but are then surprised when their governments incur the Canadian-style deficits that are the logical result.

Canada's achievements in health care have been tremendous, but to some extent we are now the victims of our own success. We have managed to provide a level and quality of care for a general population that has few parallels in the world on a case-by-case basis. But we also have to understand that our great achievement at the end of the 1960s was not to socialize health care, but to socialize health insurance. We socialized insurance, and at first that's all we did. Since that time, successive governments have had to contend with health care budgets that have always shown a marked tendency to grow as a portion of overall government spending. Health care has been the single biggest item in every Ontario provincial budget since the 1970s, when medicare was first introduced. If one looks at the level of current consumer demand, as opposed to what might be called citizen demand, it becomes apparent that health care costs will continue to grow. We are getting older. Therapies are more successful and often more expensive. Home care needs and drug care costs are exploding.

Making a distinction between consumers and citizens is important. We are all sometimes consumers of the health care system and when we are, the evidence suggests that we act in our own interest as energetically as possible. We are strong advocates on behalf of ourselves, our children, our families and our communities. We live in a society where people definitely want to express their views about care and access to care, and about the therapies and drugs available. As consumers, we drive the health care system, continually forcing improvement and demanding better quality.

As citizens, we make choices based on a broader sense of what the public interest and good are. The more public these processes become, the better off we all are. Politicians would be very happy to devolve responsibility for choices to citizens at a local level, because they want to share difficult decisions. Consumers may say "We need this now," but citizens are needed to say, "Okay, but then we have to choose between this and that."

Making choices in health care is difficult, often ethically difficult, for all parts of society, whether consumers, hospitals, doctors or communities. It is also difficult for governments, which make decisions within the broader context of how much they spend on health care in comparison to spending on everything else. It should come as no surprise that an aging baby boomer population wants more money spent on health care. Yet if we were to accede in willy-nilly fashion and transfer enormous amounts of money into the system, schools would go unfunded and child poverty would be unaddressed. We wouldn't be looking at the determinants of health in a broader fashion, or preparing for the needs of the next generation as opposed to the current one. These issues are difficult, but they are the ones politicians are elected to deal with, and they have to be resolved.

The realities of the current environment don't make it any easier to deal with these issues sensibly. Health care has become a metaphor for Canada itself in a way that is true of no other social program. In the public mind, the way we care for the ill is representative of the essential principles of Canadian social democracy. Indeed, the provisions of the Canada Health Act are so widely accepted by Canadians, and the debate on health care's future so solidly framed within the Act, that those who disagree with the Act's provisions will find it difficult to participate in the debate in an inoffensive way.

A second reality is that medicare's original definition of health care and health insurance was a very narrow one. You went to the doctor, the doctor made you better. You went to hospital and recovered or died. We now live at a time where this notion of health care is inadequate — it doesn't define wellness or well-being, and doesn't take into account current therapies that allow people to live longer with illness. Pathologies which brought life to a quick end 30 years ago can now be controlled or cured with drugs that are very successful but often very expensive. This kind of progress has completely changed our picture of wellness and illness. It also makes dealing with the costs of the system more problematic. To what extent, for example, should the health care system pay for the cost of Viagra, the new anti-impotence drug? Under the American model, private insurance pays for it and adjusts premiums accordingly. Under the Canadian model, a doctor might decide the drug improves a patient's well-being and quality of life but, in the process, we see the condition become a publicly insurable item. If we pay for it, what else don't we pay for? Or is there anything else we don't want to pay for?

I do see some opportunities in the devolution of power now taking place in health care. It may well produce the kind of citizen participation that is hard to find at the provincial and federal levels. We all know that the federal government has been systematically withdrawing support from the health care system. The provinces, in turn, have had to download the impact onto local bodies, either hospitals or, when better planned, onto regional authorities that have some real ability to determine the types and levels of care that will be provided. This could well prove to be beneficial, but only if the regional authorities have the financial resources they need.

There is a sensible way to devolve responsibility for health care, but it should not involve simply dumping onto existing structures. Too often, these structures are unable to make intelligent decisions because they are only equipped to make decisions for themselves; a hospital cannot make an intelligent decision about home care or external relocation of resources, for example. But over time, the central locus of health care decision-making will devolve to a new form of regional structure that can accommodate consensus and enact appropriate decisions, something that cannot take place at levels of provincial and national government where issues become too abstract. Instead, new types of regional health and social service authorities will have to have real power, as well as real money. Ontario's district health councils currently have neither, but other provinces are acting: Quebec, Saskatchewan and Alberta all have superior community-based systems for decision-making. The country is heading in this direction, and the central issue is not about whether difficult decisions are going to be made, but about who is best equipped to make them, and what other levels of government are best equipped to do so in turn.

I argue in a recently published book, *The Three Questions*, that our health care system is unduly bureaucratic: there are far too many people in the provincial health ministries and the federal Department of Health and Welfare. Our challenge is to take this expertise and shift it to the regional authorities, where we need good people who can make difficult decisions at the local level. The federal government's current enthusiasm about reinvolvement in health care has to be carefully channeled, or it will simply be a waste of money. We do not need federally funded pilot projects reinventing a national home care program: I can think of nothing less worthwhile than a program of this kind administered by Ottawa. What the federal govenment can do is allocate resources to provinces and their regional authorities to implement these types of programs. We need the federal government to ensure that resources are distributed relatively equally across the country and that there is equal access to ideas and innovation nationally. Ottawa should guarantee adequate resources for local decision-making in home care, study the best practices and best models, and encourage the sharing of information between regions and provinces. This is what we need a national government to do. We do not need a guilt-ridden Ottawa bureaucracy resurrecting its enthusiasm for centralized health care. Nothing could be less desirable.

The federal government might also be valuable in insuring therapeutic drugs on a national basis. Ontario brought in the Trillium Drug Plan to manage often catastrophic drug costs and based the program entirely on income and the cost of drugs. There is no reason why a similar program couldn't be funded or run on a national basis. In fact, it undoubtedly makes more sense to run income distribution-type programs from Ottawa through the federal income tax program. We could also do a better job if we had one national drug approval system rather than ten, as the bureaucratic cost of replicating the approval process ten times over is ludicrous. Approving some drugs in one province and not another is a complete waste of money and time. We ought to take steps in these areas even if it is one step at a time, and the next logical step is to implement a national catastrophic drug plan to lessen the financial impact of drug therapies on some groups of people.

The greatest single political challenge in health care today is the fact that Canadians themselves have changed. The powerful baby boomer generation is extremely consumerist and prides itself on being up-to-date and aware of new treatments. Professionals today practice in an arena wholly different from that of the past. Whereas clients or patients used to simply follow the advice of their lawyer or doctor, they now have access to an abundance of information about their condition, as well as the expert support of self-help groups and advocacy groups. The context in which decisions are made has changed completely. There is no going back on that, nor should there be; we are not going to return to a deferential world.

It should not be surprising to learn, then, that while Canadians want it all, they also want to have it universally, and on their doorstep, and at all times. The public is telling us that if they do not get what they want from the public sector, they will demand it from the private sector. This is troubling because it is a constant reminder that the cost of the collapse of the system will be borne by those least able to afford it. Accessibility to drugs is now effectively rationed by income and access to a drug plan. Home care is now rationed according to the amount of money one has. Private nurses and supplies are appearing in hospitals because the public system does not provide the level of care people feel they need. At the end of the day, the cost will be borne by those less able to pay.

I am sometimes asked if I worry about a two-tier system developing in the future. I can only respond by saying that I am troubled by the system we have today. Let there be no illusion about the level of universal access that now exists: unless we make every effort to ensure that the system retains both its high quality and its universality, we might as well write its epitaph. The resources will simply not be there to sustain the system in the way that it needs. I am not generally pessimistic, but my experiences in government have made me realize that choices are not easy. Above all else, they require a willingness to recognize that firm decisions have to be made and clear priorities set. Some of the most complex issues that we face in health care, many of which I believe we can deal with, ultimately revolve around governments' difficulties in making such choices in an atmosphere of scarcity.

If Canadians cannot recognize that "Taxes are the price we pay for civilization," as Oliver Wendell Holmes once said, Canada will continue in a direction that finds its citizens increasingly less prepared to pay what is required to sustain the public commonwealth. If that is to be the case, health care may be the last bastion of our public system to go, but go it will. Of course, there are ways of designing tax systems more efficiently, and we have to recognize the impact of taxes that are too high on our competitive position, but the simple fact remains that if we push tax levels too low, we will not be able to sustain a decent public system. Canadians will have to be prepared to pay a level of taxes higher than their neighbours in the United States, because that is what allows us to define the public system and in particular, the health care system, as something unique and distinct. If we are not willing to pay that price, or seem unwilling to pay that price, or continue to vote for politicians advocating lower taxes and a dramatically smaller public sector, then the future begins to look less bright. We can only get what we are willing to pay for.

Reconciling Political and Health Care Agendas: Three Views

Redefining Entitlement to Health Care

The Honourable Monique Bégin

To discuss the future of health care in Canada most often means discussing this country's ability to continue funding "medicare" as it is
presently formulated, and about its financial burden, rather than discussing the type of system and services Canadians are willing to support. Although I have yet to hear a satisfactory answer as to what the
optimum funding level for health care should be, in Canada or anywhere else, the fact that we have now returned to a level of total
health expenditures which places us in the medium range of OECD
countries provides us with a standard of measurement as good as any.
We have to remember that between 1985 and 1995, Canada had
increased total health care expenditures dramatically. Without getting
better services or more services, or different services, we had become
the second most expensive country in the world in terms of health
care funding. At the same time, given the world we live in today, the
tax burden of Canadians could no longer be increased and the issue
of the deficit had to be addressed.

There is little doubt that it was this decade's major cuts in federal transfer payments to the provinces, as well as the provinces' passing
on these cuts to hospitals, that forced our health care system to contemplate reform at long last. To date, these reforms have largely taken
the form of downsizing and amalgamating institutions rather than rationalization, and these processes have been put in motion very brutally.
The Canadian public has felt the cuts very deeply because, apart from
Quebec which has an established network of community health centres (CLSCs), the provinces had no alternative structures capable of
managing the transition away from hospital care into lighter (and
cheaper) community care. The infrastructure needed to complement

hospitals was simply not there when the cuts were imposed on the system.

The "content" (as John Ralston Saul put it) that our health care policy now calls for should include a plan and commonly shared approach for providing health services to Canadians. Implementing such a plan requires redefining the entitlements of Canadians to health care services. In the past, our system had been, for good and obvious reasons, heavily hospital- and physician-based, to the exclusion of forms of care delivered by other players. The Canada Health Act (1984) reasserted the same five basic principles that had driven our publicly funded "medicare" since its inception; it added monitoring and control mechanisms, but did not question the premises of a health care system synonymous with hospital beds and medical care. In my judgement, to have reopened the very definition of health care services at the time would have involved a serious risk of losing some of the federal funds that came with the Act. Politics is the art of the possible: one does what one thinks is feasible, and not much more. The Canada Health Act (1984) simply fixed the system by eliminating the financial surcharges that had crept in, regardless of origin, and it did so within the boundaries of the publicly funded "medicare" as originally defined. Dentistry, optometry, ambulance services and drugs were consequently excluded from federal public funding.

REDRAWING THE BOUNDARIES OF MEDICARE

These boundaries are no longer relevant or appropriate today, but before we can contemplate expanding them to include home care or pharmacare, we need a design of what our "medicare" should be to promote or restore the health of Canadians at the eve of a new millennium. For example, how much home care should be part of publicly funded health insurance? Exactly what do we want to include under pharmacare? In my opinion, the most pressing issue is that of home care both because it dramatically affects people in their daily lives and because it is the back door through which a two-tier system is perniciously developing in Canada. I believe that the decision not to invest in home care by some provincial governments is not just a reflection of laissez-faire attitudes, but part of a deliberate strategy to let the private sector take over as it sees fit.

A COMMON APPROACH

Once we have determined the new boundaries of publicly funded "medicare," we will need a new Canada Health Act: the only set of rules we have to let Canadians know their entitlement to health care. The five basic conditions set in the Act (universality, accessibility, comprehensiveness, portability, and non-profit public administration) still serve us well, and I submit that they should remain in place. Some are suggesting that conditions such as "affordability" or "sustainability" should be added to the Act. I find this worrisome as such concepts can too easily be used to cut services or prevent necessary expansion down the road. However, the notions of "quality care" and "safety of care" might be valid additional criteria for our publicly funded health care system. Besides reflecting on the basic conditions characterizing the system, a new Act should give to health care an up-to-date, integrated definition, covering all health professionals and the spectrum of institutions and services delivering health care.

A new common approach not only includes a legal framework, but also refers to the question of governance. Devolving power to local health authorities, as suggested by Bob Rae, will be strongly challenged and not easy to implement, especially if the duplication of roles and responsibilities remains. Regional authorities must have real decision-making and budgetary power, but they must also be made fully accountable to their home provinces through a mechanism similar to the Canada Health Act, with conditions and clear rules of the game. Devolution also raises the question of public participation. The public has never been much involved in political activities at the regional and municipal levels — think of school board elections, for example — and I do not know how to bring Canadians to participate meaningfully at the local level.

In conclusion, there are a number of questionable concepts and theories circulating these days, but the one that worries me most stems from the provincial premiers' enthusiasm for the Access paper which led to the current discussions on the "Social Union." The provinces are essentially saying that they want to enforce the Canada Health Act amongst themselves, a stance that will most likely collapse into cozy, reciprocal compromises which do not take the common good — Canadians' health — as the foremost concern. The proposal's premise that the 10 Canadian provinces are true equal partners is pure fantasy, and the whole concept presents an array of serious problems.

The Domestic and International Politics of AIDS

Dr. Mark Wainberg

Most of my colleagues in health care in Canada earn less than half of what their colleagues do in the United States, leaving Canada prone to the "brain drain" phenomenon. We have large numbers of excellent quality researchers and practitioners who can easily be lured south of the border by higher salaries and much lower taxes. This is a very important and compelling issue that Canadians will have to address well into the future.

At the same time, Canada grossly underfunds all medical research. The Medical Research Council of Canada has been fighting a constant and losing battle in this regard over the last 30 years. The Canadian government has put far less money into medical research across the board than has the American government through its National Institutes of Health. At present, the money spent in the U.S. on research into all diseases exceeds the Canadian contribution by something like six to one on a per capita basis. Canada can afford to fund far fewer research grants than the United States, and the amount of research money made available to Canadian scientists is far less than in the U.S. This situation also contributes to the "brain drain," which is bound to accelerate unless the problem is addressed soon.

The example of AIDS

My mandate as president of the International AIDS Society is to try to address international issues as they relate to HIV/AIDS. In Canada, we owe a great debt to gay and community activists who have helped to set the new agenda for our health care institutions in their work on HIV/AIDS. The activism of HIV/AIDS advocates has also set a new standard for the way our society ought to respond to disease, and has been copied with some success by people concerned with other diseases such as breast cancer, and more recently prostate cancer.

Many Canadians have objected to the high costs of drugs involved in the treatment of HIV/AIDS, approximating $15,000 a year per person. However, they should bear in mind that this is actually one of the best investments government can make, a fact recently pointed out by John McCallum, the Royal Bank of Canada's chief economist. Not only are the costs of keeping people with HIV/AIDS healthy far less than the costs of hospitalization, but doing so enables these people to remain active as taxpayers and consumers. Even if we look at the situation in strictly financial terms, we see that we come out well ahead as a society by making these drugs available. This is not to say that drug companies cannot also play a role by reducing medication costs wherever possible, but the fact is that even as things stand now, these are important investments.

Sobering comparisons

It is estimated that over 35 million people worldwide are infected by HIV. In sub-Saharan African countries such as Botswana and Zimbabwe, the HIV infection rate exceeds 40%. The proportion of young girls aged 13-17 who are infected by HIV may exceed 35% in cities like Harare, the capital of Zimbabwe. Why is this? It is because young girls are all too often forced into prostitution to support their families. Not only do we have no right to be judgmental about people's activities in situations like these, we have to make sure that we take their circumstances — what is and is not possible for them — into account in our efforts to help.

As things stand right now, the populations of certain countries in sub-Saharan Africa are expected to diminish over the next generation, and the reason for this is largely the HIV/AIDS epidemic, as so many women of child-bearing age are lost. The development of a safe and effective vaccine to protect against HIV infection still represents the world's greatest hope for stemming the tide of infection, but problems of mutability and variability are such that the development of a HIV vaccine is still many years away.

Instead, we are encouraging alternative strategies to prevent HIV infection, and an obvious one is the promotion of safe sex. Although safe sex campaigns have been under way in many countries over many years, they have not been entirely effective. The governments of far too many of the developing countries hit hardest by the HIV/AIDS epidemic simply lack the political will to conduct such campaigns. This is a good example of where western governments can help, by pressuring countries with the highest increases in AIDS to establish such programs, and we should be prepared to help finance them.

Another approach is to empower and equip women to do more to protect themselves against the virus. Women are frequently not sufficiently empowered to insist on condom usage. The problem is greatest among impoverished sex workers who may not feel able to refuse a customer who insists on not using a condom. Having to choose between feeding a family and agreeing to forego the use of a condom is a difficult decision that I do not think many Canadians have been confronted with. But as virologists and researchers on the international scene, we must acknowledge these realities and develop methods that can help women protect themselves in these circumstances. We already have vaginal foams and jellies available, but making such preventive drugs available to people in other countries will require commitments from Canadian aid agencies like CIDA and the IDRC to help prioritize research into the field of antiretroviral drugs and vaccines to a far greater extent.

Governing Health Care

Senator Lois M. Wilson

When we consider a framework for health care reform and a national pharmacare system in Canada, we first must ask whether health care in Canada today is considered an industrial commodity that is expected to run on a for-profit basis. This philosophy seems to be gaining ground, especially since saving money is a high priority for every level of government. But I contend that health care should not be for sale.

Until recently, basic health services for the population were planned, implemented, and managed by government officials or other elected officials who had no financial interest and were accountable to the public. Today, we appear to be guided by a different premise, one that favours market value as a basis for decision-making. Current practice points to an acceptance of the idea that health care is just another industrial commodity. I find it incongruous that it was the Ministry of Industry, and not the Ministry of Health, which brought the patent act Bill C-91 through cabinet. A bill concerning drugs needed by sick men, women and children was treated as a product in the same category as cars and tractors.

The services in our health care system are increasingly being financed by private interests, even though experience in related fields indicates that costs rise as the public system erodes. We are seeing our system move to privatization and a two-tier system. I am convinced that a framework for reforming health care in this country must be based on the idea that citizens have a right to participate in planning their own health care, both independently and through their elected representatives. We must not leave it to a faceless corporate sector that may have financial conflict of interests and is not accountable to the public. Recently, a conference on national approaches to pharmacare intended to explore the possibility of a universal drug plan for Canada, was attended by people, groups and businesses who had a direct financial interest in such a plan. Until very recently, such a constituency would have been highly questionable as players in this kind of planning conference. Our government is hiring private companies to accomplish specific projects, and inviting corporations to help plan, guide and administer aspects of health care that were until recently the domain of public servants, such as laundry, cleaning and food preparation.

CONFLICTING ALLEGIANCES

The most urgently felt ethical conflict for the conscientious doctor or health care professional is the erosion of the commitment to the welfare of the individual patient, which is compromised in a system where health professionals become employees. When health care professionals receive compensation from an organization, they *de facto* owe allegiance to the organizational goals they are paid to pursue. These goals may not always coincide with the needs of patients.

Our present fee-for-service system for paying doctors sometimes results in unnecessary treatment. In American-style managed care, the opposite is true and physicians are penalized for doing too much, or providing care not included in the plan. Managed care that makes cost-containment or profit-making its goal, at the expense of the actual legitimate needs of sick persons, threatens elementary ethics. It makes price, availability, accessibility, and quality of medical care into free market negotiables. And inherent in any system devised solely to accumulate profit is the temptation to abuse power. The recent scandal over the alleged cover up by Health Canada at the Hospital for Sick Children in Toronto was a signal to the public that medical research integrity can be imperiled, and intimidation brought to bear on researchers by corporate pressure. The pressure from private interests must be resisted if the system is to maintain public confidence.

We have an obligation to assume leadership and advocate reforms that will benefit the poor, the chronically ill, the aged and the handicapped, all of whom are heavy users of medical care and are most vulnerable in a market economy that favours the rich and the healthy. We should place high value on the incremental development of a fully integrated and coordinated system of health care services that are responsive to the individual's needs and choice. We must clamour for a national publicly funded universal drug plan. Many of us place a high value on the continuing — not diminishing — leadership and presence of the federal government and urge its continuing negotiations with the provinces towards an equitable agreement. But first and foremost, we have a collective responsibility to defend our capacity to resist entering into contracts with organizations whose goals are in conflict with the best interests of patients, and to uphold the moral obligation not to cooperate with any system that is injurious to patients. In the end, the kind of health care system we have reflects the kind of societal values we hold, and the kind of society we want to become.

Additional Thoughts on Citizens, Choice and Good Governance

HOW CAN WE GET CANADIANS TO PARTICIPATE IN THE HEALTH CARE DEBATE?

Linda Haverstock: Given that public policy objectives need to be met within a government's legislated lifespan of four years, and that fewer and fewer Canadians even bother to vote, how can we truly hope to engage Canadians in their health care system?

Bob Rae: The public has a great deal of difficulty becoming engaged in areas where they don't see choices, and we have to find more and more places where Canadians can discuss what the choices actually are. This is not just a matter of people demanding more of their special interests, it involves looking at the tradeoffs and compromises required. The first step is for us to recognize that there is a great deal of consensus across the country on what needs to be done. There is a surprising amount of agreement on the general areas of reform, and we have to flesh that out before we can act on it. We have to give the public a chance to really participate and get involved.

Monique Bégin: I once asked senior Cabinet colleagues why the 1976 legislation funding medicare (the *Established Program Financing Act*) was passed without a provision for enforcing its five cardinal conditions. I was told that there was such good faith at the time between the provinces and federal government when they went from cost sharing to block funding at the negotiating table, that no one thought there would ever be a problem. I got stuck with the job of setting a penalty, so now I always think of enforcement when policy changes are being discussed. The other reason I see for a strong federal role is that health care has become a metaphor for Canada: it is binding and bonding and important because it expresses common values.

Bob Rae: I am not saying there should be no federal law, in terms of research, in terms of standards, in a lot of areas, but I do not think the federal government should deny the provinces the right to play a role as well. They are the ones who are running and managing the programs on a daily basis, not the federal government. Unlike Monique Bégin, I view the social union discussion as essential. The provinces are paying 85% of the costs of health care, and it is outrageous that they should be excluded from creating inter-provincial institutions to look at how that system is going to work.

Mark Wainberg: I certainly see a need for federal leadership in research. The closeness of our country with the U.S. leads many Canadians to ask why we do medical research here at all; can't we just learn from research carried out in the U.S. and elsewhere? The fact is that highly motivated health care professionals want to do research, and want to do research in the context of the academic institutions to which they are affiliated. If they are not given the chance to carry out that research in that circumstance, then they feel a betrayal in their careers and will opt to move to the United States and other countries where research funding is more plentiful. Besides the desirability of strong academic leadership in our medical schools for its own sake, having practitioners who are also high calibre researchers is important to the ultimate delivery of health care and to the education of tomorrow's physicians. One cannot divorce research leadership from ultimate quality of clinical care.

WHAT LEVEL OF CARE ARE WE ENTITLED TO?

Audience member: When I hear talk of a "basic level of care" it sounds to me like a promise being broken at a time when I no longer have any recourse.

Monique Bégin: But we are not dealing, now, with a basic level of care. The words of the Canada Health Act are generally taken to imply entitlement to a complete health care system.

Margaret Somerville: What we might start seeing more of, though, are people with conditions such as HIV/AIDS for which the top treatment would be extremely expensive for the health care system. People who need these treatments might not find them as accessible as they think they should be. Canadians think they have a right to them, but the Canada Health Act is drafted as an entitlement, not a right, and people have no basis on which to claim the treatment.

Monique Bégin: Except a moral basis.

Margaret Somerville: But not a legal basis. Where do we draw the line for necessary care when the person who has the condition will say that everything possible is, in fact, necessary?

Mark Wainberg: In reality, we will do the best we can and try to allocate as many resources as possible, while understanding that we live in an imperfect world.

Bob Rae: I do not hear many people suggesting that what we should be offering in terms of health care is dramatically less than what people have had before, only that if we want to keep what is there, we are going to have to run it with a greater understanding of the choices and compromises being made.

Lois Wilson: And health care has to be seen in the context of other societal priorities. We have elevated the issue of our own personal health to the highest level, and I really question whether that is an ethical choice.

CHAPTER 5

Ethical Considerations in Health Care

Ethical Dilemmas in the Current Health Care Environment

Dr. Nuala Patricia Kenny

The images that spring to mind when we think about ethical dilemmas in health care are those of drama and conflict: new reproductive technologies, cloning, end-of-life care, unequal access to technology, and inadequate resources. More recently, images of patients suffering because of inadequate care, families burdened by increasing demands for care, and patients dying because of unavailable care have dominated the media and public discussion. These are not simply individual issues. Economic, political and social forces all shape this health care environment. Each of these forces contains assumptions about what values should count in decision-making. Some are explicitly acknowledged in the formulation of policy, many are implicit, but generally, the values at stake in a particular decision are not clearly identified. While we can acknowledge that policy is often a short-term political response, we must also ensure that it reflects key societal values because policy is focused on the common good. It is impossible to determine what that "common good" is when there is no public forum in which to identify commonly-held values and no clear and respectful process for prioritizing values in real decisions.

Much of the discussion and debate in health care today centres around whether there is enough money in the system. The question itself is meaningless unless we can answer, "Enough money for what?" We pay for what we value; we will scrimp, save and sacrifice for something highly valued. So before we can even begin to answer questions about funding, we need to deal with the fundamental question of what we as individuals and communities value, how we might determine priorities, and who gets to sit at the decision-making table. This is the stuff of good health policy.

History demonstrates that public policy can play a significant role in clarifying the values of a society. The Canada Health Act embodies a set of values which Canadians have understood to be important. The Canadian health care system has embodied these concepts in a special way:

> At a time when other traditional expressions of Canadian values have been placed under demonstrable stress, health and health care have increased in importance and prominence as a shared and common value. In fact the health system has always engendered strong support among Canadians. In recent years, however, its significance has broadened into symbolic terms as a defining national characteristic...
>
> Canadian underpinnings of the health care system include the premise that it ought to be government-run and not-for-profit, that money is not the primary consideration and that all are entitled — as a matter of citizenship — to equal access to quality care. This typically Canadian approach is, for many people, emblematic of a commitment to compassion, to equality of opportunity, to a sense of community and to a common purpose.[1]

There is something about a health care system that carries with it a part of the moral and ethical fibre of a nation. We recognize the health care encounter as a place of moral meaning at a time when there are few places where we can address these questions of illness, dependence and mortality. In fact, the health care system may bear too much of a burden precisely because of the vulnerability that illness brings. If we attempt to be more just, more kind, more fair and more compassionate in health care than we are in the marketplace or other areas of life, how can we hope to sustain those qualities in health care? The challenges we face in health care might be evidence of new and different values; conscious rejection of traditional values or simply an erosion of values. Without an explicit reflection on the values Canadians hold in common there can be no good judgement as to which new values to incorporate and which to reject. And certainly, without attention to values there can be no good policy.

Ethics in public policy

At a time when society was fairly homogenous and had established public values, it was assumed that these values were incorporated into policy. Because this values framework was within a shared world view, it did not have to be made explicit. In our more complex and pluralistic world, values cannot be assumed to be shared. Ethics, a discipline of philosophy which helps us identify, clarify and prioritize the values at stake in decisions and actions, has become central to good decisions. Values can be defined as enduring beliefs regarding preferable behaviors and end-states. So, for example, truthfulness is preferable to deceit and a just society is preferable to an unjust one. Formal ethics offers a rigorous method for ensuring that these and all relevant values are identified and prioritized so that practical choices can be made. This ethical analysis is then a new task and one we are still learning to do well.

Until the 1960s, ethics in health care was medical ethics. It was a virtue-based ethic which relied on the character of the moral agent, the physician, to do "the good."[2] Today, not only is society more varied and pluralistic, but health care has grown more powerful and complex. Science and technology can do great good but often at great risk and great price. A patient can die from the effects of chemotherapy even as it cures their cancer. Even the definition of death has changed in response to the scientific and technologic capabilities of respirators, defibrillators and modern transplantation techniques. The right choice is not always clear. The biologic good is not the only good taken into account. Modern bioethics developed in the 1960s as an approach to these complex value-laden decisions. The initial ethics work focused on questions of individual medical benefit, patient rights and respect for patient autonomy. Medical advances since the 1960s have reinforced the focus on individual patient benefit and on questions of individual rights to medical benefit. We are becoming increasingly aware of the inadequacy of this approach as we face more demands for greater access to more technology than ever before. The challenge we face for the next century is in public policy and organizational ethics. Canadians need to develop new approaches to health care decisions that respect individuals but also address issues of community, society and choices for the "common good."

What is the current health policy environment?

The current health policy environment is not a happy place. It is perceived as unfocused and inattentive to important values. The driving force appears to be solely economic and, in consequence, all that is seen is cutbacks, downsizing and withdrawal of services. Dollars may have been saved but not without other costs. The outcome is an environment of anger, disappointment and distrust, and a general sense of promises broken and unfair burdens imposed. This climate is rife with real ethical dilemmas where the right choice is unclear because many important values need to be considered, many benefits we would want to protect and many harms we wish to avoid. It also fosters situations where the right and good choice is clear but the ability to choose it is compromised or obstructed by the inability of "the system" to respond. This is a situation that creates the ethical distress experienced by many health care workers today.

Many Canadians believe that our health policies actually obstruct and deny care rather than provide it. For most, the goals of health care reform are not clear; the goals of the health care system itself are not always clear. Is the good to equalize health status for all Canadians or to equalize access to the health care system?[3] These are two distinct goals and until it is clear which we strive for, health policy will be vague and arbitrary at best. The current environment of rampant individualism presents a problem for health policy that seeks to promote the common good. Modern science and technology focus primarily on individual patient benefit and thereby reinforce the individualism and consumerism of our time. Demands for medical responses to human needs are unlimited. No health care system could provide all possible "benefit" to all citizens. But if potential medical benefits cannot be provided for all, how do we decide what is provided and who benefits?

To be a society means having sufficient shared values to act together in balancing respect for individuals with the common good.

The first task is to identify shared values: no easy task in a culture that cherishes diversity. Then, based on these shared values we act to balance individual benefit and common good. This balancing act has become more complicated with the medicalization of life and the professionalization of care that has characterized this last half-century. The depression survivors who created the Canadian health care system saw the need to protect individuals and families from financial disaster in the face of catastrophic disease. They shared values and a vision of the common good in the creation of Canada's health care system. The baby boomer generation, in contrast, has experienced a constant stream of medical advances and ever-expanding personal choice in treatment options. These raise a real policy dilemma in deciding the boundaries of what we consider to be medical care.[4]

The World Health Organization (WHO) defined health as a condition of total physical, social and mental well-being. This broad definition seems intuitively right, but it has been interpreted progressively as the inclusion of all social and emotional well-being in the health care arena. People seek medical relief for both angina and heartache. Policy-makers must recognize the social determinants of health but this does not mean that these determinants should be medicalized. Rather, it challenges policy-makers to create a new vision which understands the importance of equality of health status and equal access to high quality health care. Ethical dilemmas, then, occur in today's health policy environment when we are uncertain about choice or action when a number of important goods are at stake. Good policy will address these dilemmas by developing ethical decision-making processes (what is called procedural ethics) and by basing decisions on important commonly held values (substantive ethics).

PROCEDURAL ETHICS: DOING HEALTH POLICY WELL

Like justice, ethics musts not only do good but must be seen to do good; justice and fairness must be transparent. Choosing the procedures and participants is a manifestation of values. Since public policy is always for the common good, the first ethical dilemma relates to the method that will be used to deal with differences, for differences are sure to arise in public discourse. Consensus, compromise and integrity are concepts which become extremely important in deciding this common good.[5] How much can we compromise before our integrity is affected? How do we decide when consensus is not possible? How do we respect "minority" values when making public policy? The procedures we develop to respect difference are as important as the strategies for identifying common values. The methods we use to choose participants will only be developed well after serious work regarding the meaning of community representation. How will blatant conflict of interest be addressed?

In formulating public policy a number of considerations will be taken into account including: ethics (Does it correspond to our values?), politics (Is it feasible and acceptable?), and economics (Is it affordable?). A major concern for procedural ethics is how we balance these factors in the final decision. More importantly, how truthfully and openly do we identify the ultimate basis for decision. This means the value basis for policy decision must be transparent. A clear danger for procedural ethics is the use of values language when the decision is based only on political or economic values.

Balancing freedom and accountability is an important task for responsible policy in the post-Krever world. How does a society decide the balance between allowing individuals the freedom to run risks and determining the locus of accountability when the potential risk becomes realized harm? Evidence and values have been postulated as the keys to good health care and health care policy, but achieving balance here is not easy. How are conflicts decided when the importance of individual freedom is outweighed by the risk and harm to the public good? Issues such as this are central to procedural ethics but assume particular importance in the present climate.

Finally, the importance of procedural ethics in public policy demands a scrutiny of who gets to participate in the policy-making process. How do we balance the value of professional expertise with that of community input? Do patients, families, communities have another kind of expertise? What kind of education does the community need to make a good decision? What is the proper role of specific interest groups? Current moves toward regional and community boards are attempts to include broad public values into health policy. But the value base for these decisions is not always clear. These boards have generally not been given the education and support they need to develop ethical analysis in this new era of decision-making.

SUBSTANTIVE ETHICS: VALUE-BASED DECISIONS

Many ethical issues arise in specific health care decisions: Who gets access to an ICU bed? Should we discontinue life-sustaining treatment? Should we offer a new and unproven but potentially life-saving intervention? How do we choose between acute care resources and those to chronic care, rehabilitation, palliative care? The decisions we make regarding health policy form the basis and context for all these individual decisions. There are a number of serious issues we need to address before we can hope to make sense of these decisions: we need to clarify our understanding of justice, identify health care as either a commodity or a different sort of entity, and determine the proper relationship between private and public interests in health care. Canadians perceive themselves as just and fair but there are radically different conceptions of justice that come into play when we make decisions. These need to be openly discussed so that fairness is a real basis for decisions. Clearly the "natural lottery" brings differing health care needs and health status to different individuals. Traditional healthcare responded to need and operated on the principle of "rescue," but as technology brings more options, concepts like "rescue" and "need" require redefinition. Medical necessity is no longer a clear and definable concept. Before we can address specific policy questions, these fundamental issues require reflection. In trying to resolve them we will get a real sense of common values. If we find that there are sufficient shared values to address health policy for the common good, we will have courage to work through a long list of important questions:

- How will we balance the need to respond to the imperative of giving individuals a fair chance at medical benefit despite good statistical evidence of poor outcome?
- How do we balance scientific evidence and patient autonomy?

- How do we set priorities for health research, resources and personnel?
- How do we decide when a relatively small health benefit to a large number should outweigh the larger benefit to a small number i.e., disease prevention programs vs. high technology intervention?
- How do we decide who gets to the decision table? What is meaningful community participation?
- How do we balance professional expertise with community and patient expertise?
- How do we address the perceived trade-offs between quality and access to health care?
- How do we decide the appropriate balance between public and private funding?
- Is public funding distinct from public administration?
- How much do we value the Canada Health Act?

CONCLUSION

There are values embedded in the health system we have come to expect. They were values held more than a generation ago, but were key concepts in the kind of society Canada desired to be. Much has changed in Canada over the last 30 years. As the National Forum on Health concluded,

Health care is first and foremost a social good dedicated to the improvement of the health and well-being of the entire community, not a private commodity. A great deal more than individual needs and advantage is at stake. Health care reform involves the renegotiation of the social covenant defining social obligations and commitments between the government and the society and between members of the society. The nature and humaneness of the society in which current and future generations will live will depend on decisions made regarding the structure and standards of the health care system.[7]

Canadians need to reassess these values; reaffirm what endures; revise where necessary. Though never clearly articulated, the underlying values in the system that developed from the Canada Health Act appear to be: respect for the dignity of persons; caring relationships; protection of the vulnerable; service to the common good; stewardship of health care resources; and a simple system. That system was not perfect; values were not always clearly manifested within it; the rhetoric was often more noble than the practice. But something of who Canadians wished to be was present in a real way. We are left with the question: What values do we choose now, and what kind of society will they care for?

End Notes

1. National Forum on Health. "Canada Health Action: Building on the Legacy." Volume II. *Synthesis Reports and Issues Papers*. Published by the National Forum on Health, Ottawa, Ontario 1997.
2. Pellegrino, E.D., Thomasma, D.C. *For The Patient's Good: The Restoration of Beneficience in Health Care*. New York: Oxford University Press, 1988.
3. Evans, R.G., Barer, M.L., Marmor, T.R. *Why Are Some People Healthy and Others Not? The Determinants of Health of Populations*. New York: Walter de Gruyter, Inc., 1994.
4. Trappenburg, M.J. "Defining the medical sphere." *Cambridge Quarterly of Healthcare Ethics*. 1997:6:416-434.
5. Moreno, J.D. *Deciding Together: Bioethics and Moral Consensus*. New York: Oxford University Press, 1995.
6. Kenny, N.P. "Does good science make good medicine? Incorporating evidence into practice is complicated by the fact that clinical practice is as much art as science." *CMAJ* 1997;157(1):33-6.
7. National Forum on Health, op. cit.

Creating a Sound Ethical Basis for Health Care Decisions: Three Views

Tensions in Ethics Policy: the Consumer vs. the Citizen

Timothy A. Caulfield

It is becoming increasingly difficult to incorporate ethical concerns into decision-making processes and policy. This difficulty stems, in part, from the encroachment of consumer culture into the health care domain. The impact of this trend can be seen in the growing involvement of the private sector in health care. Determining the appropriate role of market forces in directing health policy remains a key debate. However, it is also one that is essentially redundant, given the post-Keynesian embrace of market forces by all Western governments over the past few decades, and the resultant movement towards debt reduction, consumer empowerment and globalization. We should persist in weighing the advantages and disadvantages of a shift toward private sector involvement in health care, but the fact is that the shift has already occurred.

The challenge that remains is to understand the present and future impact of this shift on the place of ethics in health policy development. Minimally, it seems that the momentum of change in health care has made it increasingly difficult to insert ethical concerns into policy development in a way that meaningfully counters the ethos of the consumer culture. It has also weakened government's position vis-à-vis the market. Nevertheless, I believe that government, as the voice of the citizenry, remains the only entity capable of giving a formal voice to ethically-based health policy.

LESSONS FROM BIOTECHNOLOGY

While ethical dilemmas arising from private sector influence are not yet unduly problematic in some health policy areas, they are already a central concern in the emerging field of biotechnology, where the speedy resolution of a number of ethical issues is urgently needed. For better or worse, the next hundred years have been labelled the "biotech era," and biotechnology is poised to become one of the dominant economic forces of the 21st century. It is currently one of the Canadian economy's fastest growing sectors, as seen by the fast-paced development of genetically-derived drugs, the increasing availability of genetic testing, and the implementation of cutting-edge technologies like xenotransplantation. Biotech policy will inevitably become linked, if not intimately tied, to general health policy in Canada.

Despite biotechnology's great potential to provide tremendous health care benefits, it also raises a number of explicit ethical concerns, not the least of which are fears of commodification and the premature implementation of certain services. The current genetic revolution is perhaps the most ethically scrutinized scientific initiative in history. Many governments have allocated a set percentage of their research dollars to study these concerns, and yet this ethical dialogue has barely penetrated most countries' biotech policy. Rather, when it is given voice in policy, as in Canada, what we hear is the rhetoric of consumer empowerment and consumer choice, which stresses the maintenance of consumer confidence and national competitive advantage. These are all important issues, but they do not encourage an ethical basis for health policy. Given the clinical potential of biotechnologies and the billions of dollars at stake, industry and governments do not want to get bogged down in health ethics discourse. However, while the market's invisible hand may be an ideal guide for market efficiency and even technological innovation, developing meaningful ethical health policy demands something more.

DISTINGUISHING FREEDOM FROM CHOICE

The increasing dominance of the idea of consumer choice poses a further threat to our capacity for ethical health policy. The notion of autonomy remains a dominant ethical principle of health care but the principle of individual freedom has become indistinguishable from a perceived right to be unrestrained consumers of market goods. This trend has been noted by many commentators, including Canadian constitutional scholar David Schneiderman, who notes that "in a market paradigm, citizens are seen as consumers and rights are understood as a right to consume." In health care, the original idea of autonomy has metamorphosed from a right to decide what can be done to your body to a right of access to certain treatment options.

The threat this trend poses to the formulation of ethical health policy is already apparent in the area of genetic research. Despite suggestions in consensus statements and policy documents that patient access to genetic services such as sex selection and certain forms of prenatal diagnosis should be restricted for ethical reasons, research indicates that most Canadian patients believe prenatal testing should be made available on request (Fletcher and Wertz 1994). They also believe that consumers are entitled to whatever services they can pay for out of pocket. More recent international data support the findings of Fletcher and Wertz's small Canadian survey.

The implications for health care policy are obvious. Ethical health care policies result from community involvement and sometimes require placing public good above individual desires. But as individuals increasingly view themselves as consumers, and as society encourages decision making based on a consumer perspective, broad ethical policies will become increasingly difficult to formulate. As a consumer, I may want a car that goes 130 miles per hour, but as a citizen I may vote for a reasonable speed limit that conserves gasoline and secures safer streets (B. Barber, 1998). Research shows that people make different decisions as consumers than they do as citizens. What Canadian health policy needs right now are citizens.

A COUNTERFORCE TO CONSUMERISM

Despite these powerful trends, there are measures we can take to keep ethical issues front and centre. First, a strong if not dominant government presence in health care is needed. We can be duly skeptical of government decision-making but it remains the best way to ensure broad multi-disciplinary, multi-stakeholder discourse in health policy. As citizens, we must encourage government to continue to hold the commanding heights in health care. Government in turn must find ways to engage Canadians as citizens in health policy discourse, a difficult task at best.

Second, governments should seek to foster a dialogue on ethical issues and provide a framework for the application of policy conclusions. While there are many places where ethics discourse can and should happen, government remains best able to ensure the impact of ethics at a macro policy level — something that will not come from the market. The explicit mention of ethics and law in the recent federal biotechnology strategy hints that there may be some light at the end of the tunnel. In this regard, I join Dr. Nuala Kenny in advocating the establishment of a National Ethics Commission.

Lastly, we need to recognize the tension between private and public needs that is created by our consumer culture. We may never be completely happy as both consumers and citizens; sometimes we have to choose between what we want for ourselves as consumers, and what is best for all of us.

The Ethics of Waiting

Dr. Maurice McGregor

Canada's health care system is a highly ethical system, guided by the principle that health care must be accessible to all citizens irrespective of their ability to pay. The challenge facing Canadians is to preserve this system with its ethical principles reasonably intact. If we are to do this, it is absolutely crucial that the system begin to function better. There is little doubt today among Canadians that the health care system is functioning badly; it is, some observers say, in a state of crisis. And a crisis in health care, whether real or perceived, may lead to the introduction of the profit motive in the name of efficiency. Unless we improve things quickly, dissatisfaction with the system is going to lead to reforms which may leave the ethical basis of Canadian health care in tatters.

Our health care system is malfunctioning in many areas. One of its biggest deficiencies is the amount of time users have to wait for services to which they are guaranteed universal access. A system that only provides access to services months after patients need them can justifiably be said to be in need of radical reform.

As a first step in preserving our system, it is absolutely urgent to find out if and where waiting times are excessive. There is at present little data on how long people are waiting for health services. With a few notable exceptions, the data that exist are incomplete, unstandardized and often inflated. Even a recent study reported by the Fraser Institute depends solely on the responses and perceptions of medical specialists, and only 30% of the physicians solicited responded to the study's questionnaires. However precise their responses may have been, a sample of this size cannot be assumed to be unbiased.

To be of value, such data must be utterly credible, and collected thoroughly and professionally by unbiased observers. This is an ideal task for the new discipline of technology evaluation, in which Canada has emerged as a leader. There are federal and provincial organizations skilled in this discipline that could easily provide the needed information. They would first have to identify a set of key indicators such as the time it takes to get an appointment for a specialist consultation, an angiogram, or coronary surgery and then measure actual waiting times, developing a system that regularly samples data by province, by region, by hospital, and even by doctor. Results must be comparable across the country and from year to year so that performance could be assessed in a standardized way.

In addition to finding out how long waiting times are, we must establish limits on how long is acceptable. Health care providers and consumers should work together to establish agreed limits for the duration of waiting times on both medical and social grounds — the anxiety, fear and upheaval that go with waiting. It is also absolutely necessary that the results of waiting studies be published and made widely available. Exaggeration of the situation in the media becomes less likely when a patient phoning for an appointment at the local hospital can check the validity of data. There is also less likelihood of hospitals or physicians exaggerating waiting times when such hyperbole might lead to a diversion of patients elsewhere.

Information about waiting times would also allow patients and their doctors, when picking a consultant, a hospital or a laboratory, to avoid, other things being equal, those with longer waiting times. This alone would help regulate the system by shortening queues. More important, without information of this kind, serious management of the system is just not possible. Managers cannot rely on random evidence such as angry letters to newspapers to know where the bottlenecks are. The National Forum on Health recognized the need for this type of information when it stated that, "We do not have any valid and comprehensive measures of the quality of the health care system... We must develop quality of care and patient satisfaction outcome indicators which are comparable across provinces and territories."

ELIMINATING EXCESSIVE WAITS

When looking for indicators of quality in health care, waiting times are arguably the most important single indicator, and are within our capacity to measure. Furthermore, we are perfectly capable of finding ways to eliminate them. In considering how this might be done, let us first ask why waiting times were less of a problem in the past, and why they are now getting worse.

The waiting times in question here are nearly all hospital-based, so the severity of the problem depends largely on how hospitals function, how they respond to the incentives and disincentives that affect hospital productivity. The biggest incentive to increase productivity is the desire of health workers in hospitals to care for the sick. This is a remarkably powerful force. Another incentive to productivity, sometimes overproductivity, is the way doctors are paid by fee for service. The more they do under this formula, the more they are paid, and this tends to increase a hospital's output.

The biggest disincentive to productivity is the hospital budget. These are generally based on the previous year rather than on the amount of services provided. In the past, although nominally fixed, hospital budgets have been fairly generous, and hospitals have usually been able to increase services in response to increased demand. Accordingly, waiting lists were not a major problem. However, the budget tightening of recent years has left hospitals no longer able to respond to demand. Indeed, the hospitals have been in increasing trouble for several years. It is hospital budgets that have had to absorb nearly all the increased costs of the new technologies recently introduced to the system. In spite of this, between 1975 and 1994, hospital budgets were successively reduced from about 45% to 37% of health care funding, and this before hospital closures. Most hospitals are now operating in debt, and a hospital grappling with debt simply cannot take on more procedures in response to demand. So waiting lists grow longer, and nothing can be done. Or can it?

If the real problem is indeed the fixed hospital budget, surely the budgetary system can be modified. I am not suggesting that money should simply be put back into the hospital system. This would be an expensive way of achieving our objective. There must rather be an incentive to specifically increase productivity where there is a backlog. If there is a backlog in hip replacement surgery, a hospital must be paid a bonus for each additional hip procedure. The increased output is only necessary until the backlog is eliminated. So this would entail only a short term rather than ongoing commitment of money.

In summary, the problem is not how to create an ethical basis for health care, but how to preserve our ethical system. To preserve it, it is urgent to make it function better. An index of malfunction is excessive waiting times for health services. Our first priority must be to measure these consistently across the land. Our second priority must be to eliminate them using focused fee-for-service-type reimbursements as hospitals increase their productivity in the targeted functions.

Patient Choice as an Ethical Basis for Treatment Decisions

Dr. Lesley Degner

Canada's health care system is currently facing important decisions about new developments and directions in medicare. The challenge we are confronted with today is primarily one of substance: we need ideas. I would therefore like to offer up an idea, arising from a memorable case of mine, that could be useful in informing health policy from an ethical perspective. Could patient involvement in treatment decision-making actually lead to better outcomes? In 1975, I was conducting a study on the social context for clinical decision-making which involved direct observation of treatment decision-making in 14 different health care settings in Manitoba. Observing decisions being made, and interviewing people about these events, offered me a fairly clear view of different peoples' perspectives and the underlying values that guided their decision-making.

TWO PATIENTS ASSERT THEIR WISHES

The case in question involved a young mother diagnosed with Hodgkin's disease, who failed to show up for her appointment at the cancer clinic. Instead she sent a letter to her physician. It read: "I have had six cycles of chemotherapy, and I really don't think that I can tolerate any more. You are such a nice guy I know that if I show up you will convince me to do it. So why don't we have a conversation by letter and come up with a new plan, because I just can't take this anymore." And so they began a conversation by letter. An agreement was reached and she eventually came back to the clinic. I later discussed the evolution of this arrangement with her and with her physician. It was the first time that I had seen a case where a patient had actually directed or been actively involved in treatment decision-making, and it prompted me to search out others.

A second notable case was that of a octogenarian woman who refused to have surgery despite being hospitalized with a bowel obstruction. Nine specialists were called in, and pulled out all the stops to convince her to comply. But every time a specialist came to see the woman, she would pretend she could not speak English and revert to speaking Ukrainian. Yet when I interviewed her, she spoke impeccable English. Again, I was impressed by the way in which she attempted to control decision-making around her care.

These two cases date back to the 1970s, when clinicians held several strong beliefs about patient care, one of which was that patients did not have the necessary knowledge to participate in medical decision-making. It was believed that educating patients about their condition, and encouraging them to participate in medical decision-making, would only leave them open to irreversible psychological damage if the outcomes of the chosen course were poor. While these statements may sound extremely patronizing today, at the time they were very clearly articulated in interviews with many physicians.

WHAT ROLE DO PATIENTS WANT?

The health care system needs to discover what people affected with disease think about their potential for participation in medical decision-making. We particularly need to find out whether increased participation leads to better outcomes. My colleagues and I participated in accomplishing two Winnipeg area surveys, roughly ten years apart, that questioned Winnipeggers about their views on the subject, using a very simple control preferences card set (Figure 1). In 1988 about 50% said that if they got cancer they would prefer to make all treatment decisions themselves. Data analyzed in the summer of 1998 indicates that there has been a shift in members of the public, towards preferring a collaborative role with physicians in making treatment decisions. It seems clear that when healthy people contemplate facing a life-threatening illness, they feel they would want to be intimately involved in choosing between treatment options. However, when people are actually confronted with a life-threatening illness like cancer, we hear a very different story. In a study of over 450 patients

Figure 1 *The control preferences card set*

Collaborative Role

C. I Prefer That My Doctor and I Share Responsibility for Deciding Which Treatment is Best for Me.

Active Role

B. I Prefer to Make the Final Decision About My Treatment After Seriously Considering My Doctor's Opinion.

Passive Role

D. I Prefer That My Doctor Make the Final Decision About Which Treatment Will Be Used but Seriously Consider My Opinion.

A. I Prefer To Make the Decision About Which Treatment I Will Receive.

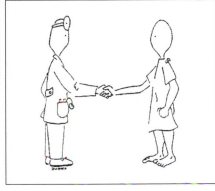

E. I Prefer To Leave All Decisions Regarding Treatment to My Doctor.

The cartoon is one of five that represent different roles in decision-making, this one being the collaborative role.
Source: *JAMA*, May 14, 1997; Vol. 277, No.18, p. 1486.

newly diagnosed with cancer, about 60% preferred to leave treatment decisions to their doctors.

But one group in the sample stood out as being committed to assuming a more active role in decision-making, and this was a small subset made up of women with breast cancer. In a study of 1,012 women, published last year in the *Journal of the American Medical Association* (JAMA), we found that in the early 1990s only about a third of the women with breast cancer in our study wanted to just "let the doctor do it." When these surveys were repeated abroad, we found that in Britain half the women were ready to leave all treatment decisions to their physicians. In Sweden, two thirds were happy to do so. Our data points to the impact of consumerism as a North American phenomenon, one that does not hold true for Western Europe.

WHAT ROLE DO PATIENTS GET?

Our findings also indicated that patients do not get to play the role they want in decision-making. Women with breast cancer only achieved their preferred roles in decision-making about half the time, and women who indicated that "keeping control" was of the utmost importance to them had only a 20% chance of assuming their desired role in decision-making. It was only those women who wanted the most passive role who had a really good chance of getting the role they wanted. What patients are telling us is that they are not being involved in decision-making, and that this is a major source of frustration to them. Consumerism is not nearly as powerful a force in health care as some would have us believe.

Men with prostate cancer seek extremely passive roles in deciding treatment, although there are indications that this is changing. Before the recent National Prostate Forum, which brought together a range of professionals and consumers, we found that 80% of men with prostate cancer stated they would prefer leaving treatment decisions to their doctor. Many of them said they would rather have their wives make decisions for them. Following that Forum, these figures began an about-face, though men with prostate cancer were still less likely than women with breast cancer to be active in treatment decision-making.

There are indications that participation in treatment decision-making benefits patients. It has been shown that patients who have been treated for a serious illness often visit family physicians for concerns related to anxiety and depression. Both our own study and others from England suggest that patients who participate in making choices about their medical treatment have lower levels of anxiety and depression, and better quality of life, for up to three years after treatment. We suspect that this translates into fewer medical visits and greater cost savings, and intend to proceed with this line of study. The idea of patient involvement in medical decisions is gaining popularity today, but when we hear people talk about how the wave of consumerism is crashing over us, we must remember that the majority of patients are still not getting the input they want in treatment decisions.

Additional Thoughts on Maintaining Ethical Practice in a Rationed Environment

ARE DOCTORS ETHICALLY BOUND TO TELL PATIENTS ABOUT TREATMENT OPTIONS THAT MAY NOT BE AVAILABLE?

Henry Dynsdale: With the advent of an evidence-based system, what the physician says to the patient about the appropriateness of certain treatments may well depend on the physician's awareness of the resources available. In my area of neurology, there is fairly good evidence suggesting that administering a particular kind of expensive treatment within the first three hours of a stroke will markedly decrease long term damage to the brain. And yet many of my neurological colleagues seem to be backing away from this sort of intervention because they are not sure that the resources required to administer the treatment are available 24 hours a day in their hospital. Should physicians alter the advice they give patients according to what resources are available?

Nuala Kenny: The Hippocratic tradition stipulates that the primary ethic of the physician is the ethic of competence. A doctor cannot do good medicine unless he or she is doing good science. They may well bring good science to a patient who, not finding it in their personal interest, rejects it. But lousy science never makes for good medicine.

One of the most profoundly serious issues that the National Forum on Health took up is that physicians do not have the information on the best treatment options they need for real time decision support. Medicine, and health care in general, has been exceedingly slow to use the information systems that are now commonplace in banking and telecommunications. At issue here is whether the primary ethic of competence to provide information for patients has become compromised and problematic.

A physician's primary obligation is still to the patient's best interest. Patients expect a physician to make treatment recommendations on this basis. One of the most serious issues for current health policy is that doctors are experienced or perceived as the people who say, "No, that's not possible," when in fact it is the system that limits resources and decides what to cover.

Maurice McGregor: Physicians have to wear two hats, but not at the same time. There is the hat of the personal physician, and the hat of the informed citizen. There is absolutely no doubt about what you do when wearing the hat of the patient's advisor. You inform your patient about everything that is relevant to his or her problem. Should doctors then go out and picket the Prime Minister's office because they do not have the resources they need to provide this care? Questionable. But this is where they should change hats and explain the issues as well-informed citizens. They will get all the attention they want from the public and the media. Our potential to guide the development of policy for our society is in no way in conflict with our duty to provide the best possible health care to the patients we treat and advise.

Timothy Caulfield: If a doctor makes a conscious decision to act in accordance with an allocation policy, rather than the legal standard of care, there may be legal and liability implications when something goes wrong. While the legal standard of care may be inflated, it is still the legal standard of care. The principle remains that a physician's primary duty to the patient is to make decisions based on the existing standards of care, regardless of any particular allocation policy. Paradoxically, Canadian law seems to be increasingly committed to enforcing this through both fiduciary and negligence law.

Lesley Degner: People are also using the media to ensure that new treatments become available. The people arriving at the emergency department are increasingly aware of the best treatment options because they have seen it on television.

Margaret Somerville: There is debate within the field of bioethics concerning the larger issue of what constitutes the full range of treatment a doctor has to disclose in order to get informed consent. The physician must reveal all material information that would be relevant to the patient, at which point the patient can make an informed decision. However, that might mean that a physician would have to tell a patient about treatments that their hospital may then refuse to provide.

RATIONING HEALTH CARE

Kevin Skilton: A number of years ago the state of Oregon implemented a rationed care plan. It was done quite explicitly, but was also paralleled with a change in state law under which physicians remained accountable and responsible for the full disclosure of treatment options to patients, but could no longer be held liable for being unable to provide care not included in the state plan. Have you noticed a similar trend in Canadian law?

Timothy Caulfield: The Oregon model is one of the few where policy makers have tried to create a liability immunity for allocation decisions. Canadian law has not followed that route, though there are so few cases that we cannot yet look at a body of jurisprudence to see a real trend. So far, the legal standard of care does not incorporate conscious allocation decisions. The courts are sensitive to and will incorporate instances of actual scarcity where resources are simply not available. But the courts have not incorporated consideration for a conscious allocation decision by a physician that puts one patient's needs over another.

Audience member: How will the rationed environment and the trend toward a consumerist approach to health care affect the commitment of our next generation of physicians?

Nuala Kenny: The young physicians of today are definitely members of the consumer generation: these are the same young people who bought $195 Reebok sneakers when they were 15. As they come into medicine today, it is fair to say that they encounter a general sense of demoralization among the older physicians they rely on as mentors and role models. And young physicians make it clear that they are not going to work the way their predecessors did. They arrive with all of the concerns of the consumer culture they come from, and are then exposed to the low morale of the previous generation of physicians at a time when opportunities for altruistic service and for estimable professional practice are fewer than they have ever been. This is a profoundly serious issue because it is these young physicians who will eventually provide the medical care of the 21st century and create the moral climate for their successors.

I want to believe Richard Cruess' optimism about the state of medical professionalism today, but I am not nearly as sanguine as he is. While doctors are often seen as advocates for individual patients, they are not seen as advocates for the common good, and therefore, have little influence on policy. And it is our own fault as doctors, because we have allowed the mechanisms through which doctors as groups deal with public policy to become dominated by a single issue: physician earnings. As a result, we have lost credibility.

Sharon Mathias: The Provincial Health Council of Alberta is a group of citizens, supported and advised by an expert panel, that monitors the progress of health care reform. The ordinary people who participate may come to address specific problems they have experienced with the health care system, but they are then empowered to become part of the larger discussion needed to build solutions. How effective do you think a forum like this can be at getting to the value issues we are facing? Or do we need a more precise methodology to approach these questions?

Nuala Kenny: I believe we are defining this methodology as we go. Policy ethics or organizational ethics (whatever you choose to call it), is a new area that we have to develop together. In Canada we can, to a much greater extent than in the U.S., create structures that more readily and directly relate to our value systems, even in a society as pluralistic as ours. Contributions from citizens' groups are crucial to efforts to ethically capture the experience of patients.

Lesley Degner: The Canadian Breast Cancer Research Initiative has been a model for stakeholder participation in directing research funds, and is now being adopted for the Prostate Cancer Initiative. Where there is very active involvement of survivors in the management committee they have brought a extremely useful new perspective.

John Ralston Saul: There is a tendency to use the ideas of consumerism and choice almost interchangeably: patients are either passive and accept advice or, because of the rise of consumerism, come in announcing that they want choices made and have an idea of what those choices might be. In fact there is passivity, and then self-interest. But there are two kinds of self-interest. One is the self-interest of consumerism, which is commercial. The other is the kind of self-interest a "citizens' forum" might represent, in which a knowledgeable public talks about self-interested choices in a way that can actually lead to disinterested activity. Consumerism never leads to disinterested activities, it just leads to Reeboks.

CHAPTER 6

Legal Considerations in Health Care

The Law's Contribution to Sound Health Policy

Dr. Bernard Dickens

Law is essentially parasitic. It depends on other people doing other things, and it reacts to them. It is therefore fitting for me, in this final chapter, to revisit issues raised in previous chapters and look at how the law confronts these issues, how some of them challenge the law, and what problems the law itself presents in creating sound health policy and ensuring sound health practices. But before getting into specifics, let me first look briefly at what law is. The law is an instrument, a tool, used by politicians through their legislative powers and declared by the courts. We are accustomed to law spelled L-A-W, but anthropologists might spell it L-O-R-E, as in folklore: both are based on complex sets of truths and fallacies that characterize a given society. This is the function of law, trying to assess what a society considers to be right and what a society considers to be wrong, a process that requires an interpretation of society, which we accept as an act of judgement and entrust to judges. The law is not immutable; as society changes, so do the interpretations of society that underpin our laws. The legal dilemmas we now face in health care are indicative of a changing society in which judgement about what is acceptable is struggling to keep pace with what is now possible.

LEGAL DEFINITIONS OF HEALTH

The concept of health is poorly managed in law. If we look at the Canada Health Act, it enables (not requires) the federal government to make payments for medically necessary care. In the same way that we have no legal definition of health, neither do we have a legal definition of medical necessity. Indeed, politicians prefer not to have a clear definition, because it allows there to be flexibility to expand the definition during good times and contract it during bad times. If we look at such documents as exist beyond Canada, such as the Constitution of the World Health Organization, we find health described as a state of complete physical, mental and social well-being. While we may balk at so broad a scope (as well as question whether such a state has ever been attained by anyone), it is clear that health constitutes much more than medical status.

If the goal of the health system is to improve people's health, we obviously have to go beyond a purely medical system and deal with education, employment, housing, nutrition, and questions of social equity. But of course this is not what the Canada Health Act provides transfer payments for; the Canada Health Act only funds medically necessary care. While we know that many medical conditions are induced by the phenomenon of poverty, poor housing, poor nutrition and poor education, attempts to improve the determinants of health take us beyond the medical system very quickly. We suppose that within the Canada Health Act the idea of necessity, though legally undefined, is concerned with survival. There are many conditions in life, such as infertility, that don't pertain to survival but affect people's enjoyment of their lives and, in that sense, their mental and social as well as physical well-being. But medically-assisted reproduction is not funded by provincial health plans because it is not necessary to survival in the narrow sense in which we interpret the Canada Health Act.

Many health-related services that are not medical per se, not necessary for survival, but that may promote health, fall outside the area of the Canada Health Act. The legal arguments used to get governments to commit resources to addressing the determinants of health arise not from the Canada Health Act but from the Canadian Charter of Rights and Freedoms, which has a provision that everyone is entitled to life, liberty and security of the person. While the Charter offers some protection against government interference with an individual's pursuit of their own health, it does not give government an affirmative mandate to furnish people with the resources needed to improve their health in this wider sense. We might look to the now 50-year-old Universal Declaration of Human Rights, but it contains no obvious enforcement mechanism for the rights it proclaims. The first challenge we face, then, is to arrive at a concept of health that includes but transcends purely medical treatment, and to give some legal substance to that definition.

BARRIERS TO ASSESSING HEALTH STATUS

Improving the health status of a population may rely more on public health research than on clinical developments. We hear more about the biotechnological triumphs of medical care, but conscientious countries also try to track the health status of their population, in a way that reflects not only surgical triumphs but also the relative purity of the water people drink and the air they breathe. Population health status recognizes that the public health environment gives us our quality of life, that a good sewer system, for example, is more relevant to health than a skilled transplant surgeon.

However, the public health field requires information and we are often reluctant to yield that information to government. There is a tremendous fear that the information may fall into the hands of those who will exploit and abuse it. The negative consequences of withholding information from those who need it to protect and improve public health tend to be less apparent.

Our laws on confidentiality and privacy represent very important and strong individual values. The Privacy Commission, along with individual activists, is extremely wary of legislation that would give government access to information on people's health status. Attempts to determine the prevalence of HIV infection in Canada have given rise to the view that government would be better for not having this information; because it could add to the vulnerability of specifically targeted groups. Specific reference to race, age, or disability is often construed as a prelude to discrimination.

This fear that specific information will lead to discrimination prevents us from looking into many legitimate questions on health factors that ought to be monitored or addressed. We cannot assess the impact of immigration from certain parts of the world on the prevalence of tropical diseases because specific questions about race will be seen as racism; we cannot easily plan to locate specialized clinics where they are most needed because we cannot ask which health problems are most pressing in a particular area without charges of discrimination. When we contemplate computerizing health data, we dwell more on the threat it presents to privacy than on the promise it offers of better care. The overriding concern with confidentiality and privacy manifest as important legal obstacles to generating the information that a competent public health service needs. Medical data remain very difficult for government to gain access to, despite the fact that we expect government to keep track of public health, to have some measure of the health circumstances of the population, and to cope with problems when they arise.

PREVENTIVE HEALTH CARE

Organized social, political, cultural, and legal systems are available to manage strategies aimed at preventing disease and injury. But the law is not always helpful in this endeavour because it must also represent other interests in society. Government attempts to control tobacco advertising, for example, have met with legal opposition on grounds of freedom of speech that has limited their success. Likewise, Parliament's attempt to tighten control of handguns has met with a very American rhetoric about accidental shootings in children being part of the price of freedom. Development in preventive health care is slow and agonizing. Legislative measures are politically resisted by those who evoke the rhetoric of freedom and economics. Educational measures rely on cooperation from established structures capable of reaching broad audiences. That cooperation is not always forthcoming.

HIV/AIDS prevention strategies have managed to overcome some of the obstacles to advertising safer sex. The television networks had no problem displaying sex in advertising, in their programs, even in the news, but when asked to run educational safe sex advertisements, they initially refused on the grounds that viewers would be offended. There is even greater resistance to the idea of teaching safer sex and reproductive health in our school system. The only preventive measure the schools will agree to teach is sexual abstinence, which is not effective in helping youths protect themselves against sexually transmitted diseases and prevent unwanted pregnancies. Failure to bring the knowledge we have to the people who can use it to good effect has had predictable consequences: between 1987 and 1994 the teenage pregnancy rate has gone up 18%; teenage girls now have the highest rate of sexually transmitted diseases of any age group, with chlamydia nine times more prevalent among 15- to 19-year-old girls than it is in the general population of Canadian women.

The most important legal barrier to using the classroom for safer-sex education has been the constitutionally protected right of the Catholic church to run its own schools. A recent decision of the Ontario court upheld this right by ruling that a denominational school system must be entitled to restrict the teaching of matters that run counter to the faith of that denomination in its schools. We will not require these schools to tell youth how to safely engage in activities that are prohibited by the church. While we can understand the basis of this ruling, it presents a challenge to preventive health strategies because it means that teaching safer sex is not going to be undertaken through the Catholic school system. In upholding the right to protect values that may warrant religious protection, the law renders the education system much less effective as a vehicle for preventive health care.

COMPENSATION FOR HEALTH RELATED INJURIES

The ongoing controversy around compensation for people infected with Hepatitis C demonstrates just how politically volatile this issue can become. When we are dealing with negligence that results in infection or injury, we want to know how that negligence will be determined when it is not admitted to. In the context of the contaminated blood supply, the government has admitted a responsibility for infections that occured between 1986 and 1990. But those infected outside that time period are also demanding compensation; not simply health services; not simply support under the social security system; but that they be awarded tens of thousands of dollars each as compensation for the injury of which they are "victims." By law, the failure to give appropriate information to patients as a precondition to their medical care is classified as negligence. That is legally actionable negligence if there was consequent damage.

Our thinking about government liability for Hepatitis C is informed by the way the legal system deals with more traditional medical liability when there is demonstrable fault. In medical malpractice law, the courts can set standards of care that influence the way care is given. For example, the requirements of informed consent have become more rigorous following a number of decisions in patients' favour, and physicians are, as a result, expected to spend more time speaking to patients and describing the options available to them.

But we also have to think about compensation in terms of resource allocation. English medical malpractice litigation was recently investigated by the Court of Appeal's leading judge, who had earlier presided over a commission looking at how the principles of civil litigation could be simplified and rendered more efficient. His findings are equally reflective, I believe, of the Canadian situation. As compared to other classes of litigation, the costs of medical malpratice litigation are disproportionately high considering the financial damages involved, particularly in low-value cases; the delay in reaching a judgement or settlement is much longer; clear-cut cases of liability are pursued and defended more vigorously and for longer times; claims have a lower success rate than other personal injury claims; and there is less cooperation between parties and more intense mutual suspicion of the adversary's motives. This is a difficult area of litigation, and if alleged negligence is met with denial, the claimant must contend with all of the problems outlined above.

What do we do when negligence is not admitted or proven? How do we deal with people infected with Hepatitis C when they were sick, needed a blood transfusion, and received the best product available at the time? Our focus is now on Hepatitis C, but we have to remember the rest of the Hepatitis alphabet. If we make the case that those infected with Hepatitis C should receive compensatory awards, what will we say to those with Hepatitis A, B and so on, not to mention those injured in other ways?

Following the Federal/Provincial/Territorial Review on Liability and Compensation Issues in Health Care, in 1990, there was a proposal to deal with medically-related injuries on a "no fault" basis, under which costs actually incurred would be paid but no extravagant awards would be made for pain and suffering. This report is only now being seriously discussed. It recommends maintaining the existing option of litigation, but providing an attractive alternative system of "no fault" recovery, under which those who could show some health-related injury would be entitled to reimbursement of proper expenses, insofar as these were not met by the provincial health plan. Lost income, retraining, renovations to make a home wheelchair accessible — those sorts of cost would be paid, and for life, but there would be no extravagant payment for pain, suffering and indignity. Interestingly, the recent commission of inquiry looking at the contaminated blood supply, chaired by Justice Krever, also recommended establishing a system of no-fault recovery, but not preserving the alternative of litigation for negligence.

These two proposals suggest means by which the legal system could be made to cope more effectively, with less friction, more entitlement, and in a sense more justice, than it does at present. The silence among our politicians on this issue is depressing. The issue of compensation is not, in fact, a legal dilemma. Lawyers and the legal system find it quite possible to accommodate this option. It is only unfortunate that we lack legal means of compelling discussion and debate among those we collectively refer to as our democratic government. Our only recourse, it would seem, is to persuade those we elect to discuss these issues and come to a decision that they will be able to explain and that will be subject to analysis and review.

Appropriate Uses of Law in Health Policy: Three Views

An Appeal to the Charter of Rights and Freedoms

Dr. Marcia Rioux

In many ways, health care has become a kind of barometer that indicates the state of the fundamental social contract of our society. The medico-legal cases with which we struggle today are not so much about medicine as they are about clarifying collective social values. Issues such as consent, confidentiality and access arise in many professional contexts, but when lives are at stake there can be no room for the expediency and compromise that characterise other types of lawsuits. Weighty moral questions must be confronted and decisions reached in the knowledge that each case sets a precedent, and each judgement tells us something about our country and ourselves.

The five principles on which the Canada Health Act is based are notions fundamental to our general sense of justice and citizenship. Health care is not, however, an area set apart from the constitutional and legal protection of individuals in Canadian law. There is a constitutional commitment to reasonable, equal access to essential services, and equitable taxation and equality before and under the law. This is the real basis for all equality rights in Canada, and these constitutional guarantees are intrinsic to the defense of equal access to treatment and the equal right to well-being. Notions of economic efficiency and evidence-based quality of practice cannot be relied upon to provide this basic guarantee; even democratic political mandates and ethical standards do not do so. Hospital ethics committees and self-regulating professions are no replacement for the Constitution.

As an absolute minimum, any health policy must conform not only to the five recognised principles of the Canada Health Act, but must also meet the standards of the constitutional guarantee of equality rights. Accordingly, we must look beyond traditional notions about standards of practice in health care to find what is truly legitimate in the field. Questions about who defines professionalism, the nature of disclosure, and the acceptable bases for determining access to scarce resources, must now be viewed in terms of the legal standards found in the Constitution and the Charter of Rights and Freedoms. These are the true legal standards of equality rights.

LEGAL STANDARDS TRY TO KEEP UP

A number of trends make this task more complicated while also making it more essential than ever. One such trend is the accelerating pace of innovation in medical technology, and the rising costs that innovation brings. Modern medical care has come to include *in vitro* fertilisation, organ transplants from animals, and the growing of human tissue in test tubes. As possibilities grow, our ability to fulfill them all diminishes, and arguments over resources become more likely. Another thorny problem is our newfound knowledge of genomics and the possibility of intervention in the actual structure of the genome. Such interventions may be seen as therapeutic in some quarters. To others they smack of eugenics. Easily available genetic information is already being used as a basis for the allocation of resources. In the United States, for example, there have been a number of legal cases where medical insurance was refused for babies with genetic anomalies the mother was aware of before birth.

There are also peculiarly singular events that can throw the practition, tradition and law of medicine into disarray. Estimates show that hundreds of millions of dollars will have to be spent to prepare the health care system for the year 2000 and the computer problems it will bring. One can only imagine the legal nightmare, comparable to the Hepatitis C blood scandal, that would result from thousands of pacemaker chips crashing simultaneously.

The other great change in recent years has been in patient awareness and attitudes. Health care consumers who were once thought of as uninformed and pliable are now knowledgeable and demanding. Newspapers are full of the latest medical advances, and patients want these new treatments for themselves, often before they are on formulary.

LOOKING FOR GUIDANCE

Where can we look for guidance in such a confusing area? We cannot isolate medical and health care from our basic social contract, as though medical ethics and law was a mysterious, exclusive domain comprehensible only to professional practitioners. Instead, we could apply existing rules of non-discrimination and human rights to health policy decisions, as we are in fact legally required to do. Doing so would launch us on what John Ralston Saul might call an integrated approach: a social imperative. It would be naive to suggest that such an approach could provide a clear map through the minefields of decision-making, but it does give us a single standard against which we can measure our health priorities both at the national level and in individual treatment decisions.

There are hopeful signs that this may already be happening. In October of 1997, the Supreme Court of Canada heard the case of Eldridge vs. British Columbia. The case concerned three deaf applicants who claimed that the legislation of the Medical and Health Services Act, which covers health care services, as well as the legislation of the Hospital Insurance Act covering hospitals, was discriminatory because it neither included sign language interpreters' services as an insured service, nor required hospitals to provide such services. These concerns had previously been considered to be more the domain of social services than health services.

The court, however, ruled that the British Columbia government had violated section 15-1 equality rights of the Charter in its implementation of the Provincial Medical Services Act. The decision was significant for several reasons. First, it articulated the court's unanimous view that government cannot escape its obligation under the Charter by delegating funds to private institutions such as hospitals. Secondly, the Eldridge decision clearly stated that in providing medically necessary services, hospitals are carrying out a specific government objective and that "the Hospital Insurance Act is not simply a mechanism to prevent hospitals from charging for their services, rather it provides for the delivery of a comprehensive social program. Hospitals are merely the vehicles the legislation has chosen to deliver the program." They cannot thereby provide services to the general public in a manner which denies some people equal benefit from the program.

Accordingly, governments and their agents, hospitals and health care providers, have a positive obligation to remove barriers that deny people the full enjoyment of the values encompassed by the health care system. The court named these values in its judgement: "The promotion of health, the prevention of illnesses and disease and the realization of those values through a publicly funded health care system."

Judgement in the Eve case of 1986 came to a similar conclusion. The case concerned the sterilisation of a young woman who could not give informed consent, and the court ruled that consent was not the issue. What mattered was the fundamental right of a woman to be able to bear children.

Medical and health care decisions are increasingly providing us with the legal cases that challenge our ethics, our policy, and our law. Health care providers alone should not be making decisions like those made in the case of Terry Urquart, a young Albertan man denied a lung transplant because he had Down's syndrome. He was finally considered for a transplant as a result of public pressure, but by then it was too late and he had died.

These types of decisions are pivotal in determining what values our society wants to adopt, uphold, and respect as we head into a new century. They are decisions about who we think is important and valuable, about who will have full citizenship rights and who will not. They are decisions grounded in notions of equality, equity, fairness and justice. It is imperative that we stop pretending that decisions of this kind are simply medical decisions to be left to specialists within health care, and regard them instead for what they truly are: decisions about the fundamental nature of our society's social contract. At the end of the day, better legal and ethical standards can only come from this kind of realization.

Moving Beyond Reactive Law

Dr. Jamie Cameron

Earlier in this collection, Bernard Dickens identified four legal dilemmas that spring from health policy, and suggested ways in which each dilemma challenged existing law. John Ralston Saul, in turn, stated that "management only works as a function or servant of policy," and went on to ask whether an emphasis on management and on the creation of additional managers actually causes more problems than it solves. As my intent here is to examine the interface between law and health care policy, I want to substitute "law" for "management" in order to ask essentially the same question.

Should law be concerned with policy, and does law cause more problems than it solves? Should the law take a leading role in questions of health policy or should it follow? Put another way, should the law simply respond when other processes have failed? Is it just a fallback, or can it be considered as a source of ideas, something that can inform and enrich health care policy?

WHEN THE LAW LEADS

These are complex questions best illustrated by example, and one of the best examples is that of the Eldridge case already raised by Marcia Rioux. In the Eldridge case, the Supreme Court of Canada ruled that it was unconstitutional for British Columbia's hospitals not to fund sign language interpretation for the hearing-impaired. Unconstitutional in this case meant that it was a violation of the supreme law of our country and its paramount guarantee of equality under the Charter of Rights and Freedoms.

The Eldridge case is seen by some as a positive example of the law leading the way, taking a leadership role and moving health care policy forward in a particular direction. Others, however, may well see this decision as an intrusion into policy-making processes, and a judicial usurpation of the roles of those who are normally responsible for making these kinds of decisions, whether it be legislatures, health care institutions, or health care professionals. The question is whether the traditional losers in the policy sweepstakes — the individuals and constituencies that don't have enough clout to count as stakeholders — should have access to a remedy that is constitutional and legal in nature. To ask why not is to recognize that certain consequences and implications attach to solutions that are generated in this way. If the need for sign-language interpretation seems self-evident, the problem is one of abstracting these issues from health care policy and resolving them through a legal analysis that is necessarily ad hoc and part of an adversarial system.

A more recent case before the Supreme Court of Canada involved an HIV-positive man who had failed to disclose his infection to partners with whom he had unprotected sex. In an especially significant decision, the court found that the man could be held criminally responsible for assault, and overturned existing assumptions about consent and fraud in finding that his behaviour could be open to criminal law sanctions. The case was particularly important because, after some debate, the court overrode the objections of interested groups who argued that such a decision could have a negative impact on AIDS testing and treatment. As a result, while there can be no doubt that criminal law is within the court's mandate, we are left with a situation where its ruling could yet have detrimental effects on health policies in relation to HIV/AIDS.

This is not to say that less law is always be a good thing. For instance, further legislation could smooth federal-provincial relations on health care policy, an overlapping jurisdiction marked by fractious relations and considerable posturing. While the tension between the appeal of national standards and the very different needs of different provinces is undeniably a political issue, we have to ask ourselves if it can only be resolved by political means. A case can surely be made for mandatory dispute-resolving mechanisms in this area.

The line between law and politics

Of course, these jurisdictional issues are far from settled. At present, we are just striking out in the dark and resolving issues on a case by case basis in an *ad hoc*, fragmented fashion. At some point we are going to have to decide where the law's jurisdiction ends and pure politics begins, a decision that will depend a great deal on who has the authority to make decisions. How that is determined remains to be seen. At stake here is nothing less than fundamental choices about who has the responsibility and the authority to make decisions about health care policy. We have not even decided what sort of decision-making process should underlie a legitimate health policy.

These questions refer to our need for a conceptual framework if we are to address difficult policy issues fairly and coherently. Until then, we will have no answers when we ask ourselves whether we should have more or less law in health care policy, and whether the law should lead policy-makers or follow them.

Litigation: A Saying-Sorry Way to Heal the Wounds

Dr. Margaret A. Somerville

Several recent developments in medical law offer some interesting insight into how the use of law in medicine reflects and affects the physician-patient relationship.

THERAPEUTIC JURISPRUDENCE
AND MEDICAL MALPRACTICE SUITS

There is a new school of legal thought emerging called therapeutic jurisprudence, which recognizes that the law, itself, has the power both to hurt and to heal, and which focuses on how we can use the law to help to heal the emotional wounds of patients and their families. Some medical malpractice suits might be examples of therapeutic jurisprudence. People who launch these suits are not always seeking compensation first and foremost. Many are motivated by the desire to publicize and stop the type of negligence that killed or injured their loved ones. The law provides the authoritative ruling that something terrible did happen, and should not be allowed to happen again. Many people experience this as some good coming out of the harm and suffering they have endured, which makes it easier to bear. They have, in a way, used the law to heal themselves.

In these lawsuits, there is always the enormous sense of a breach of trust by a professional. There is a very strong positive emotional bond that develops when patients puts their lives in someone else's hands, and if something goes wrong and the physician handles the situation badly — for instance, avoids the patient or the family — the pendulum can then swing to an equally strong negative feeling towards the physician, a feeling that many feel impelled to act upon. Here in North America, we pursue such action through the courts, as medical malpractice cases.

Fiduciary obligations

In the past, lawyers tended to think of the doctor-patient relationship as one governed by tort law or, occasionally, contract law. The contractual relationship is less frequently considered nowadays, because it is difficult to form a contract where no payment is involved. Tort law is still widely used. However, the Supreme Court of Canada is now suggesting a third way of considering the doctor-patient relationship, in which the doctor owes his or her patient fiduciary obligations. These are based on trust and mean that the physician-patient relationship is one of "the utmost confidence and good faith." This, in turn, means that the physician must never be in conflict of interest and must always place the patient's interest above his or her own interests and the interests of others.

Rights to treatment

The new type of cases we are most likely to see in our courts in the near future are those involving patients who either want certain expensive treatments that a hospital is not prepared to provide. The hospital might have guidelines that exclude patients with certain characteristics from receiving certain treatments — or want a treatment to continue when the doctor thinks no further benefit can be gained from it. If the attending physician decides or is ordered by the hospital to tell a patient they cannot have a particular therapy, in particular if the refusal is linked to reasoning that to provide the treatment would be a waste of resources, the courts will be called on to determine the limits of the hospital's power and the extent of the physician's fiduciary obligations. Among other questions, this will involve an issue of constitutional law. Article 7 of the Canadian Charter of Rights and Freedoms guarantees the right to life, liberty and security of the person, while Article 15 protects Canadians from discrimination. Provincial charters or codes of human rights legislate similar guarantees. One important question will be, what, if anything, do these guarantees in conjunction with the Canada Health Act offer Canadians in the way of a constitutional right to health care?

Additional Thoughts on Where the Law Belongs in Health Care

COMPENSATION OR ACCOUNTABILITY?

Richard Cruess: I was the only physician member of the Federal/Provincial/Territorial Review on Liability and Compensation Issues in Health Care, chaired by Robert S. Prichard in 1990, and one question we did not address was whether society uses the malpractice system as a means of winning compensation for indivduals who have been harmed or as a part of the profession's accountability system.

Jamie Cameron: Most plaintiffs who sue for compensation want acknowledgment of a mistake, some vindication of their instinct that the physician must be accountable for his or her effect on individuals' lives. It can range from a desire for punishment to a simple wish to validate their complaint. If there is no mechanism for physicians to profer an apology without running the risk of implicating themselves, then the only recourse left is the legal system. I am not convinced this serves either party well.

Bernard Dickens: The legal system also offers a means by which patients who feel ignored can get attention. They can make the doctor or hospital listen to what they have to say. It is a means of expressing their anger, their disappointment, their frustration, their sense of betrayal. The issue of seeking compensation is less pressing in Canada than in the U.S. because we have provincial health plans and a social security network.

We must remember that there are provincial variants. The Ontario health plan functions like any other insurance plan. It does not guarantee that you will not suffer misfortune, but it does say that if you do, the costs that it entails will be covered. Nevertheless, it uses the commercial practice of subrogation, where the insured is required to sue or to lend his name to suit, so that the insurer can get his money back. There are instances of litigation in Ontario that are driven and funded not by the plaintiff but by the Ontario Health Insurance Plan pursuing litigation to recoup their medical and legal costs. The Prichard recommendation was that the practice be discontinued.

Margaret Somerville: Some of the hardest policy decisions and ethical dilemmas are best handled initially by an *ad hoc*, case-by-case approach. Those individual cases then build up a body of knowledge which can help us deal with variations in later cases, and eventually allow us to come up with a policy that will encompass most situations arising from the original dilemma. Nowadays, high-profile malpractice cases are not played out solely in the courtroom, they are on national television, and provoke public discussion. Malpractice cases are one mechanism for engaging citizens in the debate. Should the law lead or follow medical practice?

Jamie Cameron: There will be cases where it is obvious the law should lead, others where it should obviously follow, and yet others where it seems best for the law to play no part at all. What we need is a set of organising principles that can tell us when there is a valid role for the law. We must decide how much legal and regulatory authority is desirable and whether there is a point at which the oversight has gone too far.

Bernard Dickens: The political system, the legislature and the courts, are in constant interaction with one another. If we find a court's decision unacceptable, we have the political power to change it through legislation. If that legislation is dysfunctional, there may be some latitude for the courts, reinforced perhaps by the Charter of Rights, to make a slightly different interpretation. If the interpretation is not acceptable, then the legislators may come back and introduce new legislation, which will again go back to the courts. Our Supreme Court, like its British and American equivalents, is not bound by its previous decisions, though political powers can put the courts' decisions into written law to discourage them from changing their minds later on.

Marcia Rioux: There have already been some very important cases where it was critical that the courts intervened because the political system failed to understand what certain practices involved and what underlying values they represented. Involuntary sterilisation was one example. The legislature ignores some issues, leaving only the courts to intervene.

Margaret Somerville: Much as physicians might hate medical malpractice litigation, it serves a very necessary function in society, and indeed in setting health policy, because it sends the strongest possible message to physicians that if they transgress ethical bounds, the law will hold them accountable. Before medical ethics was as prominent an issue as it is today, I would be invited to speak to medical students as a lawyer, because at that time they would only really prick up their ears if a lawyer said, "The judges will get you for this." We can rightly decry the harm that litigation can do, but it does serve a necessary purpose.

Bernard Dickens: Civil law is now moving towards something called "alternative dispute resolution." While recognizing that litigation is sometimes necessary, this approach contends that it is not the best way and it should not be the first way, to resolve disputes. Under our current system, if one admits fault and apologizes, this can be used to prove liability in a later suit. Health professionals faced with litigation are often advised to keep quiet and let their lawyer speak for them. On the other hand, there are cases where an apology is all the plaintiff was really looking for.

From a point of view of jurisprudence, the difficulty with alternative dispute resolution is that when you have confidential dispute resolution you cannot be sure that the same situation is being dealt with in a like manner across a range of cases, so it compromises jurisprudence — the idea that the law aims to serve the ethical principle of justice that like cases be treated alike — even if it contributes to the parties' being content.

Jamie Cameron: Any structure or institution that can promote transparency and accountability in health care relationships is, in principle, a good idea. However, the success of using an "ombudsman" approach depends very much on how it is structured institutionally, what its mandate and powers are, and how it contemplates resolving complaints and disputes between physicians and patients. Some of the alternatives to litigation now being proposed seem to be springing up by way of default. To the extent that the profession does nothing to promote its own accountability to patients or deal with issues of transparency we may well see more of these kinds of alternatives being proposed.

THE HEPATITIS C LEGACY

Margaret Somerville: There seems to be a philosophical clash between the all-or-nothing view of the law with respect to what constitutes an acceptable decision — a non-negligent one and the attempt in health policy to move towards nuanced evidence-based decisions. Everyone assumes that we proved negligence in the case of Hepatitis C, but when we went back and looked at the epidemiological evidence from that 1986-1990 period, we found that the only test available to those responsible for testing blood products had a positive predictive value of less than 30%. Had they used this test, for every ten units that would have had to be thrown out, at least seven would have had nothing wrong with them. This could well have led to a shortage of blood. Anyone working in technology assessment would say that you should never use a test with such a low positive predictive value. We are sending out very mixed messages, when we turn around and rule that they were negligent in not using the test.

We are also saying that we are not concerned about the people who got hepatitis some other way than through tainted blood. We only care that some people are very upset, and we are going to give away millions of dollars in compensation for a decision which, at the time, was the best choice that could be made. And the problem will not end with Hepatitis C. The medical community is now saying we should not do mammography on women under a certain age, or use prostate specific antigen (PSA) testing widely because the test characteristics are not very good. The whole technology assessment movement is telling us to wait until the technologies are more reliable before we use them. But we cannot wait because the Hepatitis C ruling tells us that if we do not use them, we are liable to be accused of negligence in retrospect.

Bernard Dickens: We should bear in mind that the federal ministry paid compensation over Hepatitis C in order to avoid litigation. It does not necessarily follow that if it had gone to litigation the ministry would have failed. But this is a ground on which strategically they chose not to fight. On other grounds they are willing to fight. There can be negligence in not considering a test even when the result of consideration would have been not to apply the test. And, of course, if people were not told that the test, however imperfect, was available, that failure to lay the ground-work for informed consent could also be construed as legal neg-ligence. Showing that it caused damage, however, is more prob-lematic. Legally there is no liability for making an incorrect decision, but there is liability for making a decision incorrectly. If you take into account everything that is relevant, then exercise judgement, and it goes wrong, that is considered a risk of pro-fessional decision-making and there is no legal liability for it. If on the other hand, you leave out factors that should be taken into account, or include factors that should not be, then your decision-making procedure is faulty, and that could be a source of legal liability. We are not governed only by what is scientifi-cally sound, but by what is the proper process of decision-making, even if the results of that proper process are flawed.

CONTRIBUTORS

The Honourable Monique Bégin, P.C., O.C., M.A., was the first woman from Quebec elected to the House of Commons, where she served as Minister of National Revenue and then Minister of National Health and Welfare from 1977 to 1984. She remains best known for her efforts in strengthening Canadian medicare by the Canada Health Act of 1984. Since leaving politics, Professor Bégin has served as member of the International Independent Commission on Population and Quality of Life, Dean of the Faculty of Health Sciences at the University of Ottawa, and now is Professor Emeritus at the University of Ottawa.

Jamie Cameron, Ph.D., has been a member of the Faculty of Law at Osgoode Hall Law School at York University in Toronto since 1984. Her research and teaching interests are focused on constitutional law, including American constitutional law and Canada's Charter of Rights and Freedoms. Professor Cameron is a regular participant in the public discussion of health care, especially as it relates to reproductive autonomy and access to assisted reproduction.

Timothy A. Caulfield, LL.M., is a professor of Law and has been Research Director of the Health Law Institute at the University of Alberta since 1993. He teaches law and medicine at the University of Alberta Faculty of Law, and has published numerous articles and chapters examining the interface between law, ethics and health policy. He is an editor of the *Health Law Journal* and *Health Law Review*. In September 1998, he chaired the Second International Conference on DNA Sampling: The Commercialization of Human Genetic Research.

Richard Cruess, M.D., FRS (C), was Professor of Surgery at McGill University and Chair of the Division of Orthopaedic Surgery at the Royal Victoria Hospital in Montreal before becoming Dean of the McGill Faculty of Medicine (1981-1995). Dr. Cruess is a past president of numerous professional associations, and was named a Member of the Order of Canada in 1995. Dr. Cruess and his wife, the distinguished physician and medical administrator Dr. Sylvia Cruess, stepped down from their administrative positions in 1995 to write on the subject of professionalism and medicine in contemporary society, and have presented their research both nationally and internationally.

Sylvia Cruess, M.D., was a senior physician at the Royal Victoria Hospital and is an associate professor of medecine at McGill University. She was director of the Metabolic Day Centre at the Royal Victoria Hospital prior to becoming director of professional services in 1978, serving in this capacity until 1995. She was active in the field of hospital accreditation, serving on the the body which established standards and was on the scientific advisory committee of the Canadian Broadcasting Company, and on Bell Canada's consumary advisory panel. Since 1995 she has been working with Dr. Richard Cruess on professionalism in medicine.

Raisa Deber, Ph.D., is Professor of Health Policy in the Department of Health Adminstration at the Faculty of Medicine of the University of Toronto. Professor Deber's current research centres around Canadian health policy, and medical decision making, including studying definitions of "medical necessity," examining the roles patients wish to take in making treatment decisions, and considering public and private roles in the financing and delivery of health services. She is currently president of the Canadian Health Economics Research Association (CHERA).

Lesley Degner, Ph.D., is Professor in the Faculty of Nursing, Associate Professor in Family Medicine, and Adjunct Professor in Psychology at the University of Manitoba in Winnipeg. As Nurse Scientist in Residence at Winnipeg's St. Boniface General Hospital, she advises on the integration of research into practice. Dr. Degner's primary research focuses on improving communication between cancer patients and health professionals, with a particular emphasis on clinical decision making. She is the co-author of a book entitled *Life-Death Decisions in Health Care.*

Bernard Dickens, LL.B., LL.M., Ph.D., LL.D., specializes in law and medicine, and has taught at the College of Law in London, England and Columbia University in addition to his positions as Professor in the Faculty of Law, the Faculty of Medicine and the Joint Centre for Bioethics at the University of Toronto. Professor Dickens is legal articles editor of the *Journal of Law, Medicine and Ethics*, and serves as a member of the editorial boards of several journals. Professor Dickens is a Fellow of the Royal Society of Canada, Fellow of the Royal Society of Medicine (London), Chairman of the Human Subjects Ethics Review Committee of the University of Toronto, and Chairman of the Human Subjects Research Ethics Committee of the National Research Council of Canada. In 1991-1992, he was president of the American Society of Law, Medicine and Ethics. Since 1994, he has been on the Board of Governors of the World Association for Medical Law, serving as Vice President of the Board since 1996.

Pat Kelly, former immunology researcher at Hamilton's McMaster University, is one of Canada's leading advocates for cancer patients. She is a former member of the Board of Directors of the Ontario Cancer Treatment and Research Foundation (OCTRF) and the Ontario Cancer Institute/Princess Margaret Hospital (OCL/PMH). She was awarded Canada's Governor General's Award in 1992 for her efforts on behalf of cancer patients, and was a driving force at the 1993 National Forum on Breast Cancer. In 1993, she founded PISCES

(Partners in Self-Help Community Education and Support) to serve the self-help community's needs for training and development. PISCES has conducted workshops in Canada and the United States and in 1996 sponsored the First Canada-U.S. Breast Cancer Advocacy Conference.

Sister Nuala Patricia Kenny, M.D., LL.D., FRCP(C), is nationally recognized as an educator, medical ethicist and distinguished lecturer. In 1995, she became the Founding Director of the Office of Bioethics Education and Research of the Dalhousie University Faculty of Medicine. Dr. Kenny has served on the Committees on Biomedical Ethics of the Royal College of Physicians and Surgeons of Canada and the Canadian Pediatric Society. A founding member of the National Council for Bioethics in Human Research, Dr. Kenny was part of the Tri-Council Working Group on Revision of Guidelines for Research with Human Subjects. She is a past Chair of the Values Committee of the Prime Minister's National Forum on Health, and a past President of the Canadian Pediatric Society and the Canadian Bioethics Society. She currently serves on the National Science Advisory Board.

Maurice McGregor, M.D., FRCP(C), joined the Royal Victoria Hospital and McGill University in Montreal in 1957, where he has served as Head of Cardiology, Head of Medicine, Dean and Vice Principal. From 1988 to 1994 he was President of the Conseil d'Évaluation des technologies de la santé du Québec, the Quebec provincial council evaluating health and technology and from 1994 to 1998 as Editor and Chair of the Steering Committee of the Canadian Breast Cancer Treatment Initiature. Dr. McGregor is at present Professor Emeritus in the Medical Faculty of McGill University and a senior physician at the Royal Victoria Hospital.

Devidas Menon, M.H.S.A., Ph.D., is currently Executive Director and CEO of the Institute of Pharmaco-Economics, Edmonton, and Professor of Public Health Sciences at the University of Alberta. Formerly Executive Director of the Canadian Coordinating Office for

Health Technology Assessment in Ottawa. Dr. Menon has been actively involved in health technology assessment activities at the international level, and has served on the governing boards of both the International Society of Technology Assessment in Health Care and the International Network of Agencies for Health Technology Assessment.

Terrence J. Montague, M.D., was Assistant then Associate Professor of Medicine at Dalhousie University. In 1988, he became Professor of Medicine at the University of Alberta, where he served as Director of Cardiology and as the founding Principal Investigator of the Clinical Quality Improvement Network (CQIN). In 1996, he joined Merck Frosst Canada as Executive Director of Patient Health.

The Honourable Bob Rae, B.A., LL.B., partner at the international law firm of Goodman, Philips & Vineberg, was elected eight times to the federal and Ontario parliaments during his years in public service. Premier of Ontario from 1990 to 1995, he was Leader of the New Democratic Party of Ontario from 1982 until his retirement from politics in 1996. An Adjunct Professor at the University of Toronto and an Associate Fellow of Massey College, University of Toronto, Mr. Rae is the author of numerous articles and speeches on labour and employment law, public and constitutional law, changes in the modern state, and the challenge of political leadership. His political memoir, *From Protest to Power* (1996) was followed in the Fall of 1998 by his second book, *The Three Questions: Prosperity and the Public Good.*

Marcia Hampton Rioux, Ph.D., is Member of The Graduate Program, School of Social Work at Toronto's York University and was President of the Roeher Institute, Canada's national institute for the study of public policy affecting persons with disabilities. She has consulted for the Canadian Human Rights Commission on Equality in Employment and the National Council of Welfare, and was a policy analyst for the Law Reform Commission of Canada. She is a former Director of Research for the Canadian Advisory Council on the Status of Women. She is the author of numerous articles and books on human rights and disability.

Nathalie St-Pierre, has been executive director of the Fédération nationale des associations de consommateurs du Québec (FNACQ) since 1995, where she directs research and prepares briefs on issues of privacy and the information highway, energy, biotechnology, health and insurance for presentation to government agencies, ministries and the general public.

John Ralston Saul, Ph.D., is one of Canada's most influential writers and thinkers. An internationally acclaimed novelist, essayist and social critic, Dr. Saul was variously the head of an investment bank in Paris, the assistant to Maurice Strong, Chairman of Petro Canada, and head of the Canada-China Trade Council. Dr. Saul is the author of five novels and four non-fiction works of provocative social commentary. Saul's latest book, *Reflections of a Siamese Twin: Canada at the End of the 20th Century* (1997), has been touted as "one of the best books about Canada in living memory."

Hugh Scully, M.D., C.M., M.Sc., FRCP(C), is currently Professor in Surgery and Health Administration at the Faculty of Medicine of the University of Toronto, and Senior Staff Surgeon in Cardiac Surgery at the Toronto General Hospital. Dr. Scully is President-elect of the Canadian Medical Association (CMA) beginning August 1999. He was Head of the Section of Cardiac Surgery for the Ontario Medical Association (OMA) until 1998, and a past President of the OMA. Dr. Scully is President of the Canadian Cardiovascular Society.

Margaret A. Somerville A.M., FRSC, A.V.A. (pharm.), LL.B. (hons.), D.C.L., LL.D (hons), is a Gale Professor of Law and Professor, Faculty of Medicine, McGill University, Montreal. Professor Somerville has published extensively on issues of bioethics and law, appears regularly in media and on speaking tours as an internationally recognized authority on bioethics, and is a consultant to many levels of government and NGOs regarding public policy. In 1986, Professor Somerville became the Founding Director of The McGill Centre for Medicine, Ethics and Law, created jointly by the McGill Faculties of Medicine, Law and Religious Studies. The Centre undertakes research for government, international aid agencies, and health care and medical institutions and practitioners on issues of medicine, ethics and law.

John Wade, M.D., FRCP(C), has served as Chief of Anaesthesia at the Health Sciences Centre in Winnipeg, Vice President of Medical Services at the Health Sciences Centre in Winnipeg and Dean of Medicine at the University of Manitoba. Dr. Wade served as Deputy Minister of Health in Manitoba between 1995 and 1997. He is currently Professor of Community Medicine at the University of Manitoba, as well as Chair of the Resource-Based Relative Value Schedule Commission which aims to produce a complete schedule to recommend to both the Ontario Medical Association and the Ministry of Health.

Mark Wainberg, Ph.D., is an internationally recognized scientist at the forefront of the fight against HIV/AIDS. He has made many important contributions to the study of virus-host interactions, antiviral drug development and drug resistance. The McGill University AIDS Centre, which he founded and still directs, was among the first laboratories worldwide to characterize the phenomenon of HIV escape from immunological pressure through mutagenesis. In 1989, in collaboration with BioChem Pharma Inc., Dr. Wainberg made the initial identification of 3TC, currently the world's most widely used drug in the treatment of HIV. President of the Canadian Association for HIV Research 1995-1997, Dr. Wainberg has been a member of numerous scientific and review committees in Canada, the U.S. and overseas, and is a frequent speaker at scientific meetings throughout the world. He became the President of the International AIDS Society in June, 1998.

Senator Lois M. Wilson, Ph.D., is an author, minister and internationally known authority on human rights issues. Dr. Wilson was the first Canadian President of the World Council of Churches, is the

Vice President of the Canadian Civil Liberties Association and has been Chair of the Board of the International Centre for Human Rights and Democratic Development since 1997. The author of five books and numerous articles, Dr. Wilson was made an Officer of the Order of Canada in 1984. In 1985, she was awarded the Pearson Peace Prize by the United Nations Association in Canada. In 1998, she was named to sit in Canada's Senate as an Independent Senator.